The MITCHELL Principles

A Guide to Elite Performance & A Healthy Lifestyle.

Thomas M. Mitchell DC, CCSP

Medical Disclaimer

This book contains general information about health, medical conditions and treatments. This information is not advice and should not be treated as such.

The information contained herein is provided without any representations or warranties, express or implied.

It should not be an alternative to health care advice from your physician or other licensed healthcare provider.

If you have any specific questions about any health matter, you should consult your physician or other licensed healthcare provider.

If you think you may be suffering from any health condition, you should seek immediate medical attention.

You should never delay seeking professional healthcare advice, disregard the advice or discontinue any prescribed treatment because of information contained herein.

COPYRIGHT

Contents

Intro

To my patients, *and*
To athletic directors, athletic trainers, coaches, athletes, parents of young athletes, and people just trying to live a healthier / happier lifestyle —

I WROTE THE MITCHELL PRINCIPLES SPECIFICALLY FOR YOU!

Let me keep this part short and sweet, because the important part - the meat of the matter - is beyond this short introduction.

Being athletically involved, as I have been all my life, (in sports, power lifting/weight lifting) involves training, coaching, nutrition, and sports psychology. I have realized that all of these must be learned and turned into positive habits for your athletic lifestyle to help you reach the top.

Still, as many reach for the top rung on the ladder, others stress their bodies beyond the limits established in their training. They get hurt and need help.

YES, INJURIES HAPPEN!

In my view point, it's vital to educate everyone involved, at the earliest possible opportunity, to understand this: you can get hurt and you can prevent it from happening. When injury does happen, you need to know what steps to take – to get well and dedicate yourself to future prevention efforts, so no further injuries occur.

In today's competitive sports, when you watch anything from amateur boxing, wrestling, local or national football games to an international soccer match, you'll see injuries occurring and you'll see injured athletes just pick themselves up, dust themselves off, and start all over again. In later years, they'll wonder if their 'screwed up knee' was related to the game they had in 2011. Years later, they'll often find that they need knee replacement surgery.

Here we provide a framework that will teach you how to self-manage situations that may occur.

Always remember that we are available to you at any time to be your primary contact for sports medicine and functional healthcare needs in the Chicago area. We combine injury care, prevention, nutrition, the proper management of concussion injuries, with a dynamic approach like no other provider in the region, to help you meet your health goals.

To your safe, improved athletic abilities, health and happiness,

Thomas M. Mitchell, DC, CCSP

Chapter 1

My Story

EARLY YEARS

I began weight training when I was about 12 years old. I worked very hard at it and I became proficient. Then, by my senior year in high school, I broke my first New York State High School bench press record.

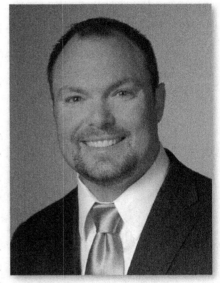

During college, I competed a few more times and I took a couple of New York State titles in bench press which made me realize how great it was to perform at such a high level.

Soon after, I realized that I wanted to go into medicine. The only problem I faced was that I really didn't know what branch of medicine would best suite my lifestyle as an athlete. After researching, I came to the realization that allopathic medicine (normal medical healthcare) wasn't me at all.

I wanted –no, I *needed* something that was involved with improving health and wellness–; not something that would restrict me to treating symptoms and prescribing drugs to those who needed medication. I needed something 180 degrees from that medical (allopathic) path. I needed a career field that allowed me to continue to expand and develop my knowledge and information base; to keep myself healthy, and live my life based on that career field while continuing to be athletically successful and win championships.

CHOOSING A CAREER FIELD

The idea of chiropractic came to mind, and after some research, it moved right up to the top of my list of medical fields to explore. In fact, my research proved to me that chiropractic medicine is a model for a medical career field in preventative health care and wellness: for keeping people healthy and active.

In my second semester in chiropractic school, when I was 22 years old, I went into a research study for performing lower back adjustments. As one of the requirements for the study, I received a free MRI. (Magnetic Resonance Imaging)

The results of the MRI examination resulted in my getting booted out of the Lumbar adjustment study because, apparently, I had several herniated lumbar discs, as well as something called Schmorls nodes*.

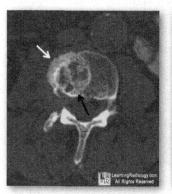 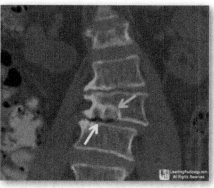

Schmorl's nodes (first described by a German pathologist, Christian G. Schmorl in 1927) are defined as herniations of the intervertebral disc through the vertebral end-plate. They are believed to be associated with trauma, especially in the thoracic and lumbar vertebrae. It is generally agreed that trauma likely precipitates the actual formation of the Schmorl's node. In the maturing spine the epiphyseal plate may represent a weak spot of annular attachment, allowing for some disc material to extrude, causing an inter-body nuclear herniation. It is now generally accepted that these nodes could predispose the disc to degenerative changes at an earlier onset, especially when observed in the earlier age groups.

Indeed, this was a big surprise to me. I didn't know how I could possibly have anything wrong with my back, because I was a power lifter and I was stronger than I'd ever been. How could this be?

I was a football player in high school and a Division 6, first team All-star on the offensive line, and I never weighed more than 165 pounds back in high school, so I had to be really strong. I also had to be fast as lightning to compete, but hearing about and understanding what Schmorls nodes were, came as a complete and total shock to me. Because I'd never been injured, it's tough to say why my lower back was in this condition, although it may have been related to participating in football and power lifting when I was younger.

On a positive note, I was impressed by the realization that I had never experienced any back pain at all. This wisdom led me to two insights that I was unaware of before:

1. A damaged spine does not have to hurt or be disabling, and

2. I'd have to reinvent my training to care for my back and keep myself healthy.

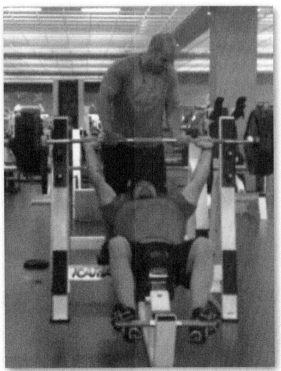

Now, 15 years later through following my own advice and learning how to naturally achieve a healthy, athletic lifestyle, I'm stronger than I've ever been I'm still pain free and still competing at a high level.

Currently I hold several national bench press records, the most recent in April of 2013. In the near future I will focus on a world record.

IN THE HEALTHCARE FIELD, WHO AM I

If I were asked 'who are you and what do you do?' I'd probably say "I'm Tom Mitchell, and I am a Natural Healthcare Practitioner, Certified Chiropractic Sports Physician, Chiropractic Physician, a Functional Rehabilitative Specialist with a certification in Applied Kinesiology as well as a proficiency in Clinical Nutrition.

Through combining Kinesiology with chiropractic adjustment expertise I have developed a reputation for my ability to produce positive results where others have either failed or achieved only partial results. My well-earned brand at the Clinic, is:

"RESULTS-DRIVEN HEALTHCARE."

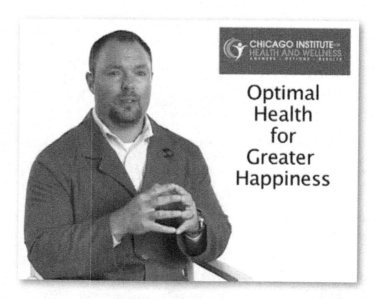

WHAT ABOUT THE IMPORTANCE OF NUTRITION

For patients who are interested in Clinical Nutrition, an in-depth introduction is available for creating a healthier diet. This nutritional program combines a modern approach to nutrition with the patient's normal daily exercise. I have many successful, long-term, enthusiasts in the "Living Healthier Family."

Every patient is unique, but everyone has similarities to some degree. Surface issues tend to run deep, and these are not necessarily resolved by using one technique alone to treat them. This is why I study, learn, test and utilize technology to help me successfully do what I do. I am dedicated to doing my absolute best—every day. I am driven by helping everyone get the best out of both their health and well-being, no matter what age, weight, or condition they are in when they begin.

Every chiropractor is unique in his or her own way, as well. We each have our particular way of doing things and our own personal skill set. Still, the greatest gift I can give is to play a role in helping others change their lives and health behaviors for the better. Doing this involves showing them the way to become pain-free and inspiring them to be healthier, more vibrant and more alive.

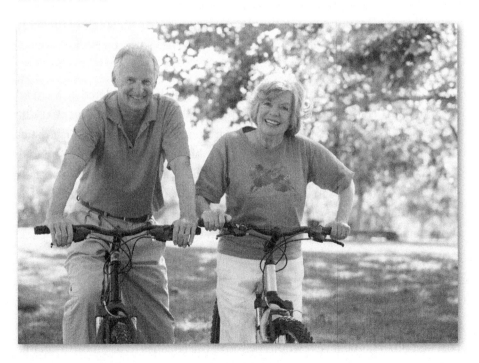

Parenting the Young Athlete

As a concerned parent, who has children that are athletically inclined, my program for young athletes is based on what I have learned, practiced, developed, modified and taught others so that the young can benefit from it. I am involved with many different organizations whose aim is helping athletes of any age achieve more with reduced risks.

I am the chairman of the American Academy of Sports Practitioners, with members integrated from various health fields including orthopedic surgeons, medical doctors, chiropractors, podiatrists, strength and conditioning coaches, athletic trainers, and massage therapists; all for the purpose of improving communications and rapport between the healing professions to help athletes receive the finest care possible.

I am also a founder and Director on the Board of The Sports Combine, an organization geared to athletically, medically and psychologically assess youthful athletes. We help young athletes get a baseline on their skills so that they can train properly to perform at a higher level. We also work on injury prevention by assessing the athlete's joints for any instability that may result in injury. If its determined that the athlete has some instability, proper rehabilitation can prevent injury.

Our group has recently created what might be considered a form of psychological testing/personality screening. When used to its potential, the screening allows athletes to be assessed for their psychological characteristics they possess that are the basis of their highest performance potential. Characteristics such as leadership, coach-ability, anxiety, mental fortitude, etc. are assessed. This screening then provides advanced guidance to help the young athlete improve or create new character skills that are beneficial for more than just the chosen sport activity. They can also create a life of excellence.

FOCUS ON PREVENTION – START EARLY

For as long as I can remember, I've always felt that, in high school or college athletics, there must be more focus on injury prevention. As one who has coached others, I believe it would behoove the coaches to use more available services to educate our young athletes. There is a great need for more health coaches trained to assess the health of athletes rather than performance coaches who are just focusing on the game. Without health coaching, young athletes can get hurt, and those injuries can last a lifetime.

Certainly a curriculum with more injury prevention (discussions, films, and materials) as well as prevention assessments of the athletes themselves would benefit any athlete or team. As it stands today, the current athletic sports physical requirement for the State of Illinois, in my opinion, is poor and far too limited in scope to be of any value in evaluating the athlete for potential injuries.

At this time, the physical examination doesn't assess instabilities in the knees, the ankles, or the integrity of the shoulders and spine. In actuality, the entire physical component of the athlete is not well evaluated at all.

Their exams do not lead to prevention of injury, but only limit the number of young athletes that might be at risk of severe asthma attacks or have heart conditions. These rarely happen, however, they are the stories that stand out in the media.

I wonder how many young athletes get hurt competing in sports compared to those that die from a heart condition after running. It must be astronomically different. Injuries on the field occur every day but deaths are rarely heard of.

Still, as of today, no injury prevention mechanisms are in place and, there still need to be more detailed assessments. Because there do not seem to be any changes happening on that front in the near future, our organizations will continue applying pressure. This is such a serious issue that it cannot be ignored.

THE SPORTS MEDICINE PATIENT

In the field of sports medicine, we evaluate and treat all types of sports injuries and achieve remarkable results. We are also one of a few professional medical clinics that provide treatment for concussions and we are extremely proud of the positive outcomes these individuals are experiencing from our care.

In our office, we see a fairly diverse set of patients with varying conditions. I see a lot of "functional medicine" patients; people that come to us to learn how to reverse health conditions such as diabetes, obesity, lack of energy, etc.

In general, overweight patients, are looking to be more physically fit, even athletic. People with hypertension are looking to reduce stress and tension and get their numbers to drop. Those who have heart disease and elevated cholesterol levels come to our clinic because they know we can assist them with changing their lifestyle to live a longer, healthy life.

THE CHALLENGE – FIND THE CAUSE

Our primary goal is to treat the cause and we often find there's some underlying chronic, inflammatory process occurring. Once we figure out what that is, we apply the approach that best suits the patient's current health status and structure the program accordingly. This includes educating the patient about the underlying issues of that condition, what the long-term ramifications are, educating them on their individual treatment plan, and holding them accountable for following the program using empirical data.

That also holds me accountable and truly, when we make those partnerships in health, the patient gets positive results and we both feel great.

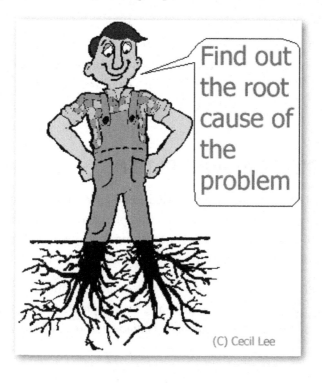

(C) Cecil Lee

Chiropractic Healthcare tends to bring up preconceived notions of what chiropractors actually do. It's amazing, that when I begin to describe the service in my practice, patients' eyes often grow wide. Obviously, they had no idea what a chiropractor really does.

I SOLVED THAT PROBLEM

Simply by writing this book, I've made this knowledge and the plan available to help people make a shift in consciousness and gain some understanding of what chiropractors do, and specifically what I do to help my patients.

As far as my personal experience goes, I can unequivocally say that Chiropractic Medicine is the finest profession in the healthcare industry. Chiropractors are trained to have extensive knowledge of the human body and are forced to figure things out without the aid of pharmaceutical medications (pills) to conceal and suppress symptoms.

Although this may sound like a hardship, it isn't. In fact, it forces us to figure out the right thing to do to get patients better naturally. We can't prescribe a drug to reduce the symptoms, so if the patient is going to get better under our care, we need to get to the root cause of the disease or impairment, and…

PREVENT IT FROM HAPPENING AGAIN

There's a preventative and functional wellness element to what a properly trained chiropractor can and will do for you during your treatment. This might include discussions and education regarding functional nutrition and training about how to perform certain movements and exercises for increased flexibility during strenuous activity.

It is well known in the world of chiropractic that 80% of patients will get better with the traditional chiropractic care, spinal adjustments. Many chiropractors promote themselves as headache, neck and back pain specialists and they follow the 80/10/10 rule, 80% of their patients get better, 10% remain the same and 10% get worse. That makes things easy for the chiropractor to do his job. The 80% that get better, give referrals and the other 20%? Well, that's just the nature of their practice.

Now, 80% success rate is a huge testament to the power of spinal manipulation. It really does work, it's just that it doesn't work for everybody. So what do you do to help the other 20% that don't get better? Well, that's where a more holistic approach comes into play.

Just to define "holistic", what I am discussing the assessment of the person as a whole, not just the spine and the nervous system.

I focus on achieving results for each and every patient that walks through my doors. Although, I do spinal adjustments, 80% is not "good enough" for me or my patients. We have to create strategies and employ all the tools necessary to help that person. I focus on getting every patient better and if I can't do it, them my job is to get them where they need to be to get better, even if it means referring them to someone else.

MINE IS A SUPERVISORY ROLE

When you're into supervising care, it's hard work, and it takes a great deal of time, energy and effort to ensure that the patient improves, whether they're a triathlete, a baseball pitcher, a football player or a 42-year old mom with four kids who is hypertensive. It doesn't matter who the patient is - it's essential to supervise the care. As holistic physicians we are given a puzzle in pieces and we must examine all the pieces, implement a workable solution, and then, when health is restored, we've solved the puzzle. As a part of this process, I add a wellness component to my work with patients and especially athletes. This is why understanding human nutritional, requirements is so vital and why my focus on how the human body works is so essential to my patient care process.

HOW PATIENT EDUCATION HELPS

I teach my patients, from the time they first enter my office, that our protocol includes patient education about what is going on with them, how we'll treat their situation or condition and why. That first day we discuss what they can expect over the period of time encompassing their treatments and office visits.

Normally we'll start with a thorough consultation that includes a comprehensive physical examination with a report of findings. I go over all of the objective data and tests in considerable detail with each patient, so the time I counsel the patient involves a highly personalized educational process based on what is going on with their bodies specifically. And it's definitely not *"your blood work shows your uric acid is high, take this pill and I'll see you in 6 months"* type of healthcare.

WHEN PATIENTS UNDERSTAND, THEY COOPERATE

When patients understand what's happening to their bodies, they usually get a clear-cut idea of why I am providing education and therapy. I'm asking them to cooperate, by participating - whether it's for rehabilitation, dietary change, increase of activity, decrease of activity to some degree, or whatever might be required for their betterment.

When they don't understand what's wrong, or your theory behind the treatment, then what you'll discover is that they've agreed to comply with something they really don't understand – and the lack of compliance occurs at remarkable speed.

COMPLIANCE IS MANDATORY

Once compliance is lost, the loss of positive results soon follows … and that is simply not acceptable. So, I educate my patients through a one-on-one sit down and make sure that they understand their health situation and what's occurring. I make sure to enlist their agreement to comply with the program in order to help my patients help themselves.

To achieve that end, I tell every patient, "any time you need a question answered, just stop and ask the question, and make sure I answer it to your complete satisfaction, because if you're uncomfortable with the answers that you're getting, you're in the wrong place."

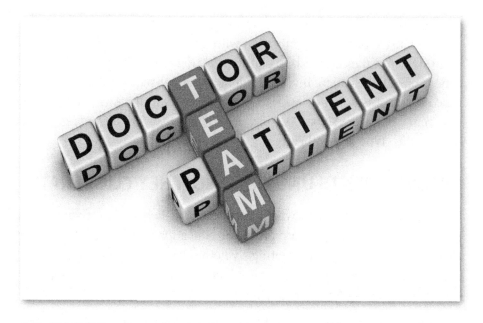

BE SMART - PARTNER WITH YOUR HEALTH CARE PROFESSIONAL

In a physician-based partnership with a patient, use objective medical reports and results as data to:

- Guide
- Evaluate and
- Address the treatment of medical issues that have already occurred

And, doing that naturally leads to:

- Decreased Healing times
- Health Body Composition
- Reversal or elimination fo functional metabolic conditions
- Overall Healthier People

This partnership relationship is so beneficial to those who are very active – including athletes and sports professionals. The true goal is health, well-being and achieving improvements in strength and energy which will show up as increased ability and performance.

Helping the athlete and patient achieve greater strength, energy, and stability is included in their overall improvement process and helps them learn how to prevent injury. Everyone benefits from this discovery including me, the physician. Once again, I will confirm that everyone who wants to be healthier will know how to reach that goal if they will partner with me and agree to comply fully with the program.

I call this process of working together with the athlete (or any other patient) Health Coaching. The partnership you form with your Health Coach will guarantee that you will achieve your *athletic* goals by learning how to achieve your *health* goals.

So if this is what you desire:

MAKE THE DECISION

"I want to live healthier."

Remember,

Habit is the key to all permanence. It's not magic. It's lifestyle.

Chapter 2

Injury Prevention

Ben Franklin once said,

"An ounce of prevention is worth a pound of cure,"

From my viewpoint as a Chiropractic Physician who sees injuries daily, I think that statement is extraordinarily accurate. Wouldn't you rather know how to prevent an injury than to deal with one after the fact, when you are in pain and suffering?

Whatever your answer is, do not worry. This book will take care of both situations. Here we'll consider it all; from food to form and function. We'll help you in every way, to put it all together for both the athletically inclined *and* for those who just want to get healthier.

Let's analyze what's required to prevent injuries in different situations.

The risk of injury will be significantly reduced by completing an effective warm up consisting of exercises that increase your heart rate and get your pulse up, followed by sport-specific, dynamic stretches (stretches while moving).

To further reduce the risk of injury:

- Eat correctly for your body and your sport!
- Apply Neuro-Stabilization Training.
- Receive proper coaching.
- Take at least 1 day off per week from your particular sport activity to permit the body to recover from the stresses.

- Use the right gear. You need to wear proper protective equipment such as pads (neck, shoulder, elbow, chest, knee, shin), helmets, mouthpieces, face guards, protective cups, and/or eyewear. This is basic, and younger <u>athletes</u> shouldn't believe that <u>protective gear</u> protects them from performing dangerous or unwise activities. *Nothing protects us from our own stupidity when we show off to others.*

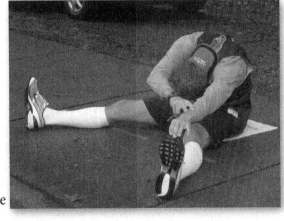

- Build your muscles. Performing conditioning exercises before games and during practice strengthens your muscles that get stressed during the game.

- Improve your overall flexibility. Stretches before and after games or practices tend to benefit your body by increasing flexibility.

- Use proper playing technique. This must be reinforced during the playing season and coaches must enforce this for player longevity.

- Take breaks. Your body needs rest periods during practice and during games. These will reduce injuries and prevent heat illnesses.

- Follow safety rules. Certain sports have 'rules' for safety including no headfirst sliding (softball and baseball), spearing (football), and body checking (ice hockey).

- Avoid injuries from heat by drinking plenty of fluids before, during and after exercise or games.

- Decrease or stop practices or competitions during high heat/ humidity periods.

- Wear light clothing during brutally hot weather.

- And, above all, **stop the activity if there is pain.**

Prevention is something that all athletes can grasp. No one wants to get hurt: of course not. But no one can guarantee that reading this book will ever stop you from getting hurt. What will happen (hopefully) is that you will learn how to take care of yourself if you do get hurt and maybe how to make sure it doesn't ever happen again. No matter what sport, activity or walk of life you work in, I think we can all agree on preparedness and care as beneficial toward prevention.

Together, in the next few chapters, we'll go discuss proper diet, training, coaching, technique, mental preparation and - most importantly- how to put it all together. It might not solve all your problems, and it is not a recipe for effortless success, but with a little reading and some hard work it will get you on the right track.

From there, I'll talk about injury care, treatment options and what chiropractic medicine does. First, let me start by saying:

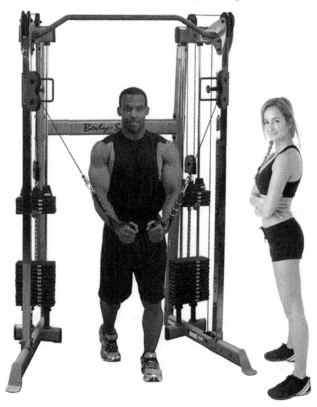

Injuries Occur

Unfortunately, no matter how hard we try, sometimes we get hurt. Be it from overuse (usually seen in the arms and upper body) or as a sudden ballistic injury (usually occurring in the legs and overall lower body), all injuries need to be properly cared for. Back injuries are particularly delicate and can be either related to overuse or ballistic injury.

INJURY VS. SORENESS

The first thing that you must understand is that there is a significant difference between an injury and physical soreness. As soreness is common, usually something you will feel directly *after* exercising, being in a game, or some other strenuous activity, you must become aware of what soreness feels like. It's very different from an injury.

Injuries, on the other hand, are usually felt *during an event* and can hinder you from doing whatever you are doing, even after the event. If you are injured, when you try to resume normal workouts or game play, the damaged tissue continues to stress during any activity and you typically feel it at that time. The muscle or tissue becomes inflamed and that is something that you will notice as swelling in that part of your body. You will probably feel tenderness or a feeling of warmth to the touch.

Obviously, you're not expected to be an expert on injury, but to know the difference between being sore and getting injured is something you must be able to determine. If you determine that you are injured you must go to an expert for help. In the meantime, be extremely cautious! If you can't recognize the difference between soreness and injury get yourself to an expert quickly to determine if you are sore or injured.

Please hear me clearly — I'm not saying that all nicks and dings that can occur whenever you are practicing or playing any particular sport need "medical" attention. But, injuries that go untreated can become lifelong issues. Rather than take chances with a lingering pain or discomfort from an injury, go see an expert.

WHAT CAUSES AN INJURY

Many things can. If you watch team sports you'll have the opportunity to see, first hand, lots of injuries occurring. Unless you have instant replay, sometimes it isn't exactly clear how a specific injury occurs. Other times we can easily trace the cause and discover what exactly went wrong.

In the best-case scenario, we pray that no one gets hurt. Regretfully, that's not always the case, and in the next chapter we'll begin to discuss what happens when someone does get hurt. For now, let's talk about how to avoid being injured.

USING SPORTS AND EXERCISE TO BUILD STAMINA

If you are a newbie, planning to use sports to build stamina, or participating in a rigorous exercise program to build up your body strength, no matter what your age, here is some information you need to know. These are basic preventive measures to help you avoid injuries through warm ups, routine fitness check ups and stamina-building exercises.

To begin with you need:

1. A Routine Physical Fitness Test -

Before beginning any new program, you should always consult your functional sports medicine doctor first and foremost. Usually, the human body tends to react negatively to any new activity, and when the activity is forced, it creates a stress on the body and sometimes results in injury. In talking with your doctor, you can go into your own personal health history to hopefully reduce the risk of injury. Depending on your age and physical condition, a stress test may be required.

Have a "True" athletic physical assessment to assess any risk of potential injury. This is required because you must modify your sports exercise and body building programs according to your current health condition. Your doctor will advise you on how to set your limits and suggest not only the right exercise for you, but also tell you the stress level that your body can endure under your particular fitness regimen.

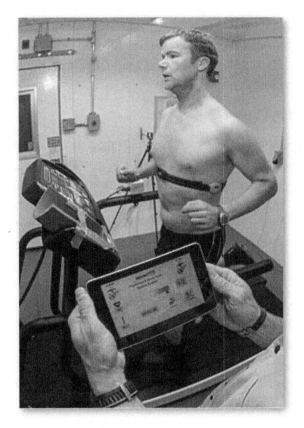

2. Increase your physical activity in phases.

After you've been cleared by your doctor, this is the second most important concept to understand. All too often many beginning athletes, with lots of enthusiasm, overexert themselves with vigorous exercising and develop fatigue from over exertion that they aren't yet ready for. You wouldn't ask a small child to carry something too heavy for them, would you? Then why push yourself into physical activity you're not yet ready for? Participation in sports is not a one-day camp event nor is it the buzzer round of a quiz competition. You're not going to walk on to a field or into a gym the first day and work like a pro. You must *build* to that strength level. When people participate in this mad rush and over-enthusiastic approach they often seriously hurt themselves.

The wise approach is to start with warm-ups and stretches, as mentioned earlier, and start with moderate exercises for 20 minutes at the beginning, then work out three times a week and gradually build the tempo based on this initial, slow momentum.

3. Never work out on an empty stomach.

It's a really bad practice to exercise or participate in vigorous sports immediately after having a heavy or moderately heavy meal. Just as they told you not to go swimming after eating when you were a child, similarly no sports or exercises should be undertaken on an empty stomach. You must eat at least two hours before playing the sport or working out. This will help you maintain the adequate energy levels that are required to exercise and avoid fatigue during the workout and during sports performance.

4. Drink Water Before You Exercise.

Dehydration is a great killer of personal enthusiasm and performance. Therefore, keep your body well hydrated. Drink at least 16 oz. of purified water two hours before you start your workout or your game, and drink water during your exercise or sports and performance to replenish the fluids lost during the exertion.

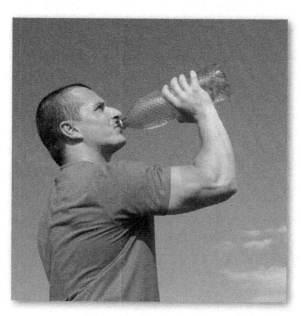

5. Listen to Your Body As It Speaks to You.

If you experience any weakness, sharp pain or light-headedness while exercising or playing, do not ignore these symptoms. Pay proper attention to them. These signals are your body's way of telling you that something is going wrong and you should take action immediately. If you ignore these warnings, that's a sure way to develop severe and chronic problems and injuries. When you do not feel well, you should rest until your body recovers. If the body sends these signals repeatedly, get to your doctor right away.

6. Rest and Recover.

It is important to rest. Sleep is one of the best ways to recover your body's energy level, but sleep alone might not be enough for some people with less stamina. If they work out too much for too long, it can lead to overtraining syndrome and possibly harm the body, by reducing the body's immunity, instead of benefiting it.

7. Cross Train w/ Neuro-stabilization.

Human beings have a creative mindset. If they are asked to do the same work every day, they ultimately get bored. Similarly, people who perform the same exercises every day are prone to develop 'workout boredom'. The best remedy for this is cross-training. It provides a complete workout for your body without overstressing certain muscle groups.

8. Wear the right gear for the specific sport.

You don't wear workout sweats while going to a black-tie party, do you? No way! People would think you were nuts if you did! In the same way, wearing the proper sports gear and footwear is essential to prevent injuries as well as wearing the appropriate safety equipment, as advised by your coach or trainer. The proper gear is designed to protect from you from accidental injuries.

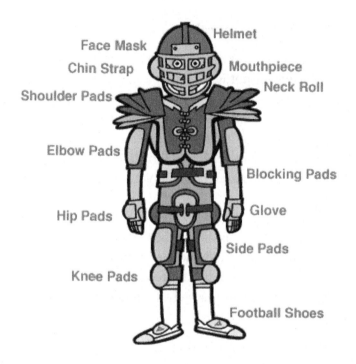

An example of protective gear

SPORTS INJURIES & PREVENTION

Whether you are a young adult brimming with the natural exuberance, vigor and vitality of your youth or a bit older and simply trying to maintain fitness, you must understand the negative consequences of negligence while involved with sports and exertion.

If you've watched competitive sports, injuries are as common as the joy of winning the game. Injuries co-exist with all types of competitive games. Even a martial arts master, like Jackie Chan, has undergone several surgeries due to the injuries he sustained while performing dangerous Kung Fu maneuvers.

You are no Jackie Chan but perhaps you are a beginner in learning about sports as a path to gain better health, goals. The old saying goes, "The winds and waves are always on the side of the ablest navigator," and at times you will be at the receiving end of playing sports, i.e. getting battered, and sometimes you might get injured.

Sports are physical activities characterized by great exertion, that must be approached under the supervision of an expert such as a coach or trainer, who knows not only about sports but also the potential of associated physical injuries as well.

I'm sure many of you might love different sports as they entertain or inspire you to become more physically fit yourself so, I've listed some of most popular sports along with the most common injuries related to them and how these injuries can be prevented. Each sport has it's own set of unique injuries that are associated, however the basics of prevention are very similar, as we discussed earlier in this chapter.

1. Baseball –Common Injuries

This is a very popular game not only in the United States but also in many other countries. Baseball is a sport that demands speed and force. Thus, this game has the highest rate of related injuries. As early as 2010, more than 40,000 players were treated in hospitals for baseball related injuries, and more than 50% were 18 years old or younger.

Common types of injuries in baseball are:

- Cuts & bruises.
- Shoulder injuries
- Back injuries
- Muscle pulls, also called strains.
- Ligament injuries or sprains.

As I said earlier, baseball is a highly spirited game in which players run, jump, skid, throw and swing their arms and legs. Players can bump into each other while running or catching. Thus, the chances of sustaining both contact and non-contact injuries are very high.

HOW TO PREVENT BASEBALL INJURIES

There are two sides to the prevention of baseball injuries. Both coaches and players have to do their respective part in the prevention of injury.

1. It is essential that coaches have a basic understanding of first aid, emergency awareness, and thorough field knowledge.

2. Players should warm-up before the match and must undergo pre- season sports medical examinations to eliminate any doubt regarding their health and fitness. Similarly, they should wear all the protective gear, not only during the games, but also while practicing.

Beyond these mentioned items, there are other safety precautions to take, such as inspecting the ground for uneven surfaces and debris strewn on the field, using breakaway bases, etc. This responsibility belongs to the management, coaches, trainers, and their staff.

Preventing baseball injuries should also include limiting the use of young players, particularly those who tend to go overboard out of sheer enthusiasm. Overuse might take many forms such as playing for multiple teams in one season, pitching on successive days, etc.

The bottom line is that you should never neglect the signals from your body. Pay attention so that sports health professionals can take care of the injuries immediately.

2. Cheerleading –Common Injuries

Cheerleading is definitely a sport and is closely associated to many other sports. It is a strenuous physical activity that combines acrobatics and gymnastic moves, which stress the body.

There was a sad incident that happened to a cheerleader in March, 2006. A young girl named Kristi Yamaoka, a student of Southern Illinois University, had a near-fatal fall from atop a human pyramid and sustained multiple vertebral fractures and internal damage in major organs. Fortunately, Kristi had a good recovery; it was a relief for everyone whose attention was focused on her during her treatment.

65% OF THE INJURIES SUSTAINED BY ALL FEMALE STUDENTS ARE INFLICTED DURING CHEERLEADING ACROBATICS.

Cheerleading involves potentially dangerous performances that are akin to stunts, i.e. forming multi-level human pyramids, somersaults, etc. Hence, the chances of injuring joints, bones, skin, etc. are very high, and Kristi's incident shows that internal organs can suffer damage as well. Head, neck, vertebra, disk, and lower body injuries are all quite common in cheerleading.

HOW TO PREVENT CHEERLEADING INJURIES

For school age cheerleaders and sports players, the American Academy of Pediatrics has issued new guidelines to prevent cheerleading injuries. Now, coaches, school authorities, cheerleaders and their parents, as well as youthful players must adhere to these guidelines. Below are the main preventive measures suggested by AAP.

- Cheerleaders must be provided with qualified coaches and medical staff.
- They must undergo pre-season physical and stamina building exercises conducted by qualified staff.
- Stunts and pyramids must be formed on a soft floor like foam, spring or grass.
- Pyramids must not be formed more than two floor levels, i.e. over two persons' height.
- If any cheerleader is exposed to an injury, he or she can only be allowed back into the cheerleading activity with a clearance certificate from a medical expert.

There are specific and detailed guidelines for pyramid formations: the base supporter should *stand* still in direct contact with the floor, and the suspended cheerleaders should never rotate, invert or dismount from their positions carelessly. Similarly, when a cheerleader is tossed up in the air (flyer), at least four players should be attending to the flyer. The flyer is advised not to drop his/her head lower than the horizontal plane with his/her torso.

3. Gymnastics –Common Injuries

Perhaps you've watched the Olympic gymnasts perform, when you were younger, and you were indeed bewildered by the sight of them bending their bodies like Elastic Woman, and perhaps you grew up wishing to become a gymnast like Nadia Comaneci, who was the first female gymnast to score a perfect 10.

Although I appreciate your aspiration to become the world's best gymnast, I also wish to share some of the hard facts about injuries associated with this sport, as well as measures to keep you safe.

Gymnastics is a sport where the gymnast develops great physical and emotional fatigue. The physical stresses are rigorous and intense, and the psychological stress is enormous as the players always want to achieve the perfect 10 for every competitive performance.

In gymnastics, athletes use the upper part of the body: elbows, shoulders and wrists more than other body parts. Hence, injuries associated to these body parts are recurrent. Some of the common injuries are:

- Elbow dislocation
- Wrist sprains
- Shoulder injuries like Superior Labrum Anterior Posterior lesions (SLAP), etc.

There are also injuries associated with the lower body such as:

- Lower back injuries
- Achilles tendon injuries
- Foot and ankle injuries

HOW TO PREVENT GYMNASTIC INJURIES

- Prepare yourself appropriately, following your coach's guidelines and advice.
- Avoid dehydration, as it can increase the body temperature, which leads to further injuries.
- Maintain both on-season and off-season fitness.

- Scale up gradually towards complex gymnastics. No need to hurry yourself.

- Warm up and cool down at every practice and event These are most important to avert many of the most common gymnastic injuries.

These are most important to avert many of the most common gymnastic injuries.

Additional preventative measures include wearing protective gear, taking breaks when you have any pain, and also checking equipment before using it.

4. Ice Hockey –Common Injuries

Hockey is a game where players use their sticks to gain control over a puck while skating on ice. Because of the fluidity of the sport and the level of impact to the player when checking or being checked by another player, the level of injuries can be substantial.

Hockey has two varients - field hockey and ice hockey - and there are specific injuries associated with each one. For the purposes of this book, I am talking mainly about ice hockey.

As hockey is an intensive game that involves skating, maneuvering, checking, and other dangerous plays, players should use specific protective gear.

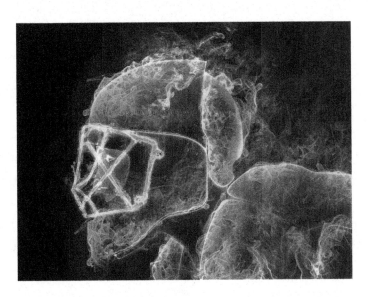

Commonly occurring ice hockey injuries are:

- Facial injuries
- Hand and wrist injuries
- Knee and ankle injuries
- Back Injuries
- Concussions
- Injuries related to overuse

HOW TO PREVENT ICE HOCKEY INJURIES

Choose the right gear. There are different kinds of protective gear for a player and the goalkeeper.

Use cardiovascular and strength building exercises to help your body withstand the physical toil and avoid quick fatigue or weakness, which can cause injuries due to falling or slipping

Improve your maneuvering skills and flexibility before playing an amateur or professional game so that you can avoid injury while on the ice.

Strengthen the neuromuscular regions of knees and ankles, and perform the necessary training under the supervision of a good strength and conditioning coach.

These are common tips, but you can learn and adopt many other tips from coaches and senior players.

5. Martial Arts –Common Injuries

Martial arts precede the world's most ancient of sports. They have been widely practiced in Eastern civilizations around China and Japan for thousands of years. In the past 100 years, they have gained popularity in every part of the world for self-defense and competition.

There are many variants of martial arts like Tae Kwon Do, Kung Fu, Judo, Karate, etc. Some of them do not involve any equipment at all, but others involve the use of weaponry like swords, knives, and other implements specifically designed to cause pain and injury.

Martial arts commonly involve utilizing high energy levels and vigorous body movements. Speed is one of the most critical elements of participating in martial arts because surprising the enemy is the goal.

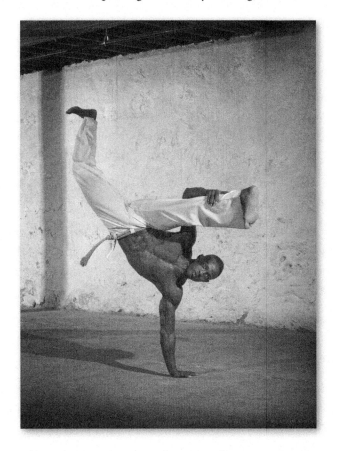

Intensive participation in martial arts tends to consume a great deal of bodily resources, causing fatigue and exertion. This can often lead to nausea, dizziness, headache, etc.

The most common physical injuries are in the skin, knees, wrists, fingers, head and extremities. Strains and sprains are quite common among martial arts practitioners. Fractures and dislocations can also occur when the player loses his/her focus, and can occur due to overuse as well.

HOW TO PREVENT MARTIAL ARTS INJURIES

- Seek advice from your family doctor before participating in martial arts classes.
- Do not attempt to practice when you are undergoing medical treatment.
- Warm up for at least 15 minutes before you flex the muscles.
- Never overuse the body parts.
- Be careful while using weapons. You have a long way to go before you are as good as Bruce Lee with weapons.
- Relax fully and allow your body to cool down after training.

You must bear in mind that the rules of martial arts should never be violated as they are meant to protect you from many negative effects. So, follow the rules and protect yourself.

6. Volleyball –Common Injuries

Invented in 1895, this game has taken the sporting world by storm within its first century celebrations. According to statistics published by volleyball.org, in the US alone more than 46 million people are playing this game, and over 800 million all over the world.

The unique aspect of volleyball is that it involves many overhead movements as the players have to do a lot of blocking and spiking. Players are constantly moving and have to use wrists and fingers extensively.

Injuries in volleyball players are commonly in the neck, shoulders, back, wrists and fingers. Volleyball players can also sustain foot and ankle injuries. Fingers are the most affected, as players do a lot of digging and setting.

Injuries can be fractures, dislocations, ligament and tendon tears. Ankle sprains and Patellar tendonitis (inflammation of tendon) are the other commonly occurring injuries. Volleyball players often develop low back pain due to the heavy use of muscles and ligaments.

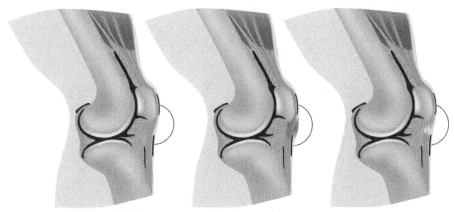

Patellar tendon intact   Patellar tendon inflammation   Patellar tendon degeneration

HOW TO PREVENT VOLLEYBALL INJURIES

- Focus on strengthening the lower back, legs and shoulders before playing the game.
- Wear ankle taping to prevent your ankle from rolling over.
- Do not unnecessarily jump on hard surfaces.
- Never stretch yourself when you are in pain.
- Remember that warming up and cooling down the body is essential.

Football – Common Injuries

No discussion of sports would be complete without mentioning football. Professional, American football as it is played today, developed from the sport of rugby in the late eighteen hundreds. It's one of the most popular sports played by young athletes from "pee wee" and high school to college and professional leagues. Football is also the leader in the number of injuries sustained by its players. In 2007, more than 920,000 athletes under the age of 18 were treated in emergency rooms, doctors' offices, and clinics for football-related injuries, according to the U.S. Consumer Product Safety Commission.

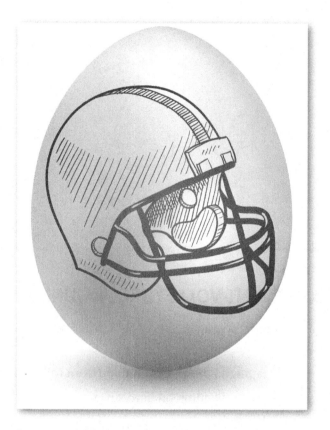

The combination of high speed partnered with full contact creates many opportunities for serious injury during football practices and games. Regardless of all the protective equipment, football players are prone to injury anywhere on their bodies. Common examples of these are:

- Knee injuries (especially those to the ACL - anterior cruciate ligament)
- Ankle sprains due to the surfaces played on and cutting motions
- Shoulder injuries
- Concussions
- Low-back pain, or back pain in general
- Heat injuries (a major concern for youth football players, especially at the start of summer training camp when some of the highest temperatures and humidity of the year occur)

HOW TO PREVENT FOOTBALL INJURIES

- Have a true pre-season health and wellness evaluation
- Perform proper warm-up and cool-down routines
- Consistently incorporate strength training and stretching
- Stay hydrated adequately to maintain health and minimize cramps
- Maintain muscle tone and strength training during summer break to prepare for return to sports in the fall
- Wear properly fitted, protective equipment
- Tackle with the head up and do not lead with the helmet

Soccer- Common Injuries

The original "futbol" is known as soccer. Historical evidence shows that a game very similar to our present day version of soccer has been played in various cultures, from China to ancient Greece, for over 3000 years. With over 3.5 billion fans worldwide, soccer is the most popular sport on the planet, according to wiki.answers.com. This international popularity has also made soccer the fastest growing team sport in the United States. This sport provides a great aerobic workout; helps develop balance, agility, coordination, and teamwork. Soccer players of all ages must be aware of the risks for injury. Injury prevention, early detection, and proper treatment can keep kids and adults on the field for many years.

Due to the tremendous amount of running, twisting and turning on foot, injuries to the lower extremities are the most common in soccer. These injuries may be traumatic, such as a kick to the leg or a twist to the knee, or result from overuse of a muscle, tendon, or bone. Most frequently, we see:

- Sprains and strains of the knee and ankle
- Cartilage tears and ACL (anterior cruciate ligament)
- Over-use injuries (Shin splints, patellar tendonitis and Achilles tendonitis)
- Stress fractures (occur when the bone becomes weak from overuse. It is often difficult to distinguish stress fractures from soft tissue injury.)

- Wrist sprains, wrist fractures, and shoulder dislocations (especially in the position of goalie, from reaching and falling on the ball)
- Injuries to the head, neck, and face (cuts and bruises, fractures and neck sprains from collisions with other players)
- Concussions

HOW TO PREVENT SOCCER INJURIES

- Have a pre-season physical examination and follow your doctor's recommendations
- Use well-fitting cleats and shin guards
- Be aware of poor field conditions that can increase injury rates
- Use properly sized synthetic balls — leather balls that can become waterlogged and heavy and are more dangerous, especially when heading
- Inspect and secure mobile goals that can fall on players (request fixed goals whenever possible)
- Drink plenty of fluids to replace those lost through perspiration and intense exertion
- Pay attention to environmental/weather conditions, especially in relation to excessively hot and humid weather, to help avoid heat exhaustion
- Maintain proper fitness (including the off-season) through activities such as aerobic conditioning, strength training, and agility training.
- Avoid overuse and over-training injuries. Listen to your body and decrease training time and intensity if pain or discomfort develops.

In other sports the injuries are to the skull so we have included an entire chapter on the treatment of concussions, as this is an evaluation and treatment specialty of our clinic. Prevention is the key to stop concussions from occurring.

PROFESSIONAL ASSISTANCE FOR PREVENTING SPORTS INJURIES

Professional help is vital in health matters. Once health is lost it's very difficult to get it back. The work involved to regain health is much harder than a steady diet of exercise, practice, preparation and prevention.

The information provided in this book includes my highest recommendations for you to avoid injury through prevention and learning how to care for yourself, should you ever get injured.

Now I'd like to take it to the next level by incorporating nutrition, neuro-stabilization training and proper pre-season athletic assessments into the mix.

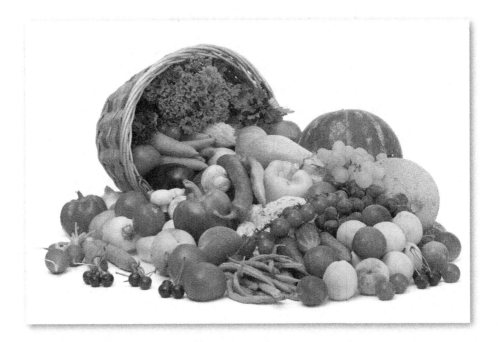

Nutrition:

As I will mention later on, in the chapter "Sports Nutrition", make sure that you eat the right foods. It's far more critical than you know. If you don't have the right nutrients to perform your energy levels will be low, and you may sustain an injury. If you don't have the proper nutrition, it will be more difficult for you to recover after exercise or injury. If you get hurt and your nutrition doesn't feed your cellular structure, the tissue can't be repaired and that may lead to a whole slew of other problems. If the tissue doesn't heal properly, it can't perform at its optimum, and optimum performance is what you strive for in your sports involvement.

Then, when you try to push yourself through your routine exercises, like you always would, you might end up hurting yourself. Damaged tissue is an injury. When it comes to food, getting what you need, and getting it at the right time, in the right form, can help you avoid injury. If you do get hurt, the right food can help in the reparation of damaged tissues.

DON'T NEGLECT YOUR NUTRITION

In general, food is often neglected or overlooked when, in fact, it should be the cornerstone of your routine. As an athlete, your body requires certain nutrients so that it can be prepared to perform at its best. That being said, don't ever go out and grab the first diet/nutrition plan you see.

Everybody is different and so are athletes. What works for one may not work for another. I believe that having a customized nutritional program is your best bet to ensure that it's tailored to your specific needs and your particular sport involvement.

Often poor nutrition is the cause of injury, and this type of injury doesn't go away all by itself. These are the injuries that linger and you may never feel the same again if you don't take proper action. Injury can also lead to chronic inflammation, which results in further injuries that your body can't repair properly.

Just as there are professional services available to help you prevent sports-related injuries through proper nutrition there are other services available to help assess an athlete's potential in order to know where they stand before they go out and perform. This is what we call a "True Base Line Athletic Assessment".

True-Baseline Athletic Assessment

COMPUTERIZED CONCUSSION BASELINE TESTING
Reason: To adequately assess the athlete's cognitive capabilities

FUNCTIONAL NEUROLOGICAL TESTING
Reason: To adequately assess the athlete's Neuro-functional abilities, such as:

- **Balance**
- **Proprioception**
- **Vestibulo-occular reflexes**

FUNCTIONAL ORTHOPEDIC TESTING
Reason: To adequately assess the structural integrity of the athlete's muscles, bones and joints.

Chapter 3

Injury Care

It's sad to say that injuries do happen. Previously, we've discussed how to prevent them from occurring, but what can you do about it if/when they do happen? Now, we will talk about what occurs and how to deal with an injury it happens to you.

IMMEDIATE INSTRUCTIONS, IF INJURED

1: If you get injured, **STOP PLAYING IMMEDIATELY!** This is an extremely simple concept that those who get injured can put into action immediately and easily. "Suck it up" and "Walk it off" are not good strategies for caring for an injury.

2: The acronym RICE will help you remember what to do and in what order: RICE stands for: Rest it, Ice it, Compress it, and Elevate it. This is the gold standard in the athletic training world. *Just to be clear: the 'I' in RICE stands for ICE, NOT heating pads and hot tubs.* I would also like to add the letter "S" for the word "Support" to this acronym, as in the various support devices that help to stabilize the area. But, I believe the acronym RICES seems a bit strange and not as catchy for anyone to remember.

3: Seek out a health care professional or injury specialist. In this day and age it may be as simple as walking to the sideline. Many teams now have athletic trainers and coaches on staff that can handle the evaluation and, on occasion, care for some injuries.

Side note: Athletic trainers do not receive the respect that they deserve. They are the top of the food chain when it comes to the evaluation of acute injuries, and they are often placed in difficult situations. They sometimes make life-altering judgment calls in a matter of seconds, and they, for the most part,

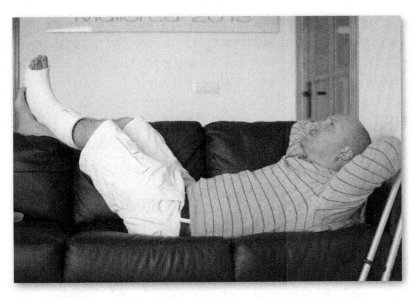

do one heck of a great job. It is easy to criticize when you see an injury the next day in the comfort of a clinic, and the treatment plan and/or diagnosis might change, but that takes nothing away from what the trainer did for urgent care. I have tremendous respect for what they do!

4: Let your body heal! Jump back into the game too early because you feel "OK" and you will quickly learn what a second or secondary injury feels like. A complete healing cycle must occur for the injury to heal properly. This process can be accelerated but only through the help of a professional who treats injuries.

5: <u>DO WHAT YOU ARE TOLD</u>! I do not go to my tax accountant to receive tax advice and then flush that advice down the toilet and do whatever I want. In sports, this behavior can get you seriously injured. If you have recommendations from a professional, listen and implement the advice, including:

- Take the necessary time off to heal,
- Follow the treatment protocol diligently,
- Follow the rehabilitation plan to get yourself back to being able to perform and take responsibility for your health.

6. Acute injuries can become chronic, and chronic injuries are the most prevalent cause of diminished sports performance. Decreased performance leads to the demise of the athlete. Then you get to talk about what you used to be able to do and not what you are now doing.

GENERAL CHIROPRACTIC CARE

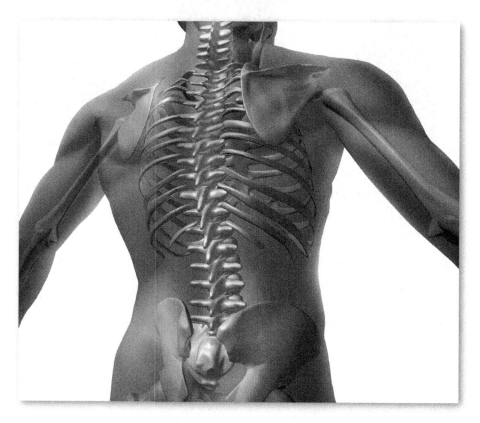

A sports chiropractor can be very useful to an athlete and a great compliment to the teams' coaches. Chiropractors know the mechanics of the body. They also benefit the athlete because they are on the wellness and preventative side of healthcare, and that's non-reactive. Non-reactive means they try to discover ways to prevent injuries, as opposed to just dealing with the injuries once the damage has occurred. A sports chiropractor can treat an ankle sprain or a torn rotator cuff, and they can also help athletes prevent them from occurring in the future.

Orthopedic surgeons, osteopathic or medical doctors in general, will typically see the athlete after the injury occurs, and the therapies are very different than that of a chiropractor. Often, a chiropractor will take a conservative perspective from both sides of the fence, for prevention and healing the damage. This methodology leads to assisting patients, athletes and non-athletes alike, in living healthier, more productive, more efficient, and more effective lives in general without the use of pain medication or surgery. *Surgery should always be considered the therapy of "last resort" when everything else has failed.*

STRUCTURAL ISSUES

When treating structural conditions, my first goal is the elimination of the patient's pain, however, just getting the patient out of pain is not the end goal. The end goal is to be fully functional, and to be fully functional an integrated approach is absolutely necessary. I recommend the following for all conditions:

- A Non-Invasive <u>Comprehensive</u> History & Examination
- Progressive Objective Testing
- An Individualized Structural Health Care Program

These may include any or all of the following in various combinations:

- Chiropractic Care
- Functional Neurology
- Health Coaching
- Physical Therapy
- Massage Therapy
- Functional Exercise Therapy
- Physiologic Modalities

The ultimate goal of implementing these essential strategies is the reversal or elimination of problematic structural and functional conditions.

STRUCTURAL CONDITIONS CASE STUDY

A 44-year-old gentleman, who had knee surgery about three months earlier was still suffering from chronic knee issues. He went to physical therapy, had his normal strengthening and stretching routines, but appropriate proprioceptive rehab was never established for him. During this time the gentleman was wearing orthotic devices.

Orthotics are customized foot devices that slip into the shoe allowing the foot to function and transfer energy throughout the system. There's something called the kinetic chain, which starts at the base of the heel, or the back of the heel during heel strike, and actually ends at the opposite base of the skull, and that's why we cross-crawl when we walk, it's the way energy transfers through our bodies as we walk or run.

When an orthotic is necessary, it allows the individual to transfer that energy correctly, so there's no abnormal stress on the joints as they walk, run or stand.

The orthotics were never reassessed after the knee surgery. The first step was to bring him in, reassess him, rebuild proper orthotics if needed, and give him an appropriate rehabilitation protocol.

You must make certain you reset the neurologic control around the knee, and make sure it's solidified through appropriate training.

Two weeks later after evaluation and treatment he's pain free, with no complications from the surgery.

CHICAGO INSTITUTE FOR HEALTH & WELLNESS

The Chicago Institute for Health and Wellness is a multidimensional clinic that offers personalized medicine. Whether it is sports medicine or functional medicine, everyone is an individual with individual issues. This is the way we treat patients within the institute. We utilize a multitude of assessment tools and treatment options to create the best care for that patient walking through our doors.

At our offices, we partner with other healthcare professionals and coordinate care within the clinic. We have specialists who will come in to treat patients individually or in groups. We have found that using a holistic approach, including treatment plans based on education and the integration of a healthier lifestyle, is most effective for our patients. Patients who are motivated to change and be healthier through their own efforts are always supported by our clinical staff. These patients are the ones that gain the most significant and positive results.

One common approach that I use is a therapeutic chiropractic treatment called a "spinal manipulation or a "chiropractic adjustment." The purpose of the manipulation is to restore joint mobility by manually applying a controlled force into joints that have become hypo-mobile, or extremely restricted in their movements, as a result of a tissue injury to the body.

TISSUE INJURY TO THE BODY

Many patients tend to sustain this type of tissue injury. It can be from a sports injury, such as improper lifting of weights, or one that occurs through repetitive stresses, such as sitting in an awkward position with poor spinal posture while performing work duties or by improperly going through a sports training. In any case, injured tissues undergo physical and chemical changes that can cause inflammation, pain and diminished function for the sufferer, all in a short period of time, and can last indefinitely if not properly treated.

Spinal manipulation, or chiropractic adjustment, of the affected joint and tissues, begins the process of restoring mobility, thereby alleviating pain and muscle tightness. This process permits tissues to heal naturally.

SCARED OF AN ADJUSTMENT

Sometimes, first-time patients are a little nervous about getting an adjustment. They soon discover that it rarely causes any discomfort at all. In fact, it makes them feel much better almost immediately – at least for the majority of patients. On rare occasions, they might feel a mild sense of soreness, like an aching, following treatment. This is similar to how someone feels after an intense workout and this feeling usually fades within 12 hours or so.

At my clinic, I have a number of patients who come in with lower-back pain. Chiropractic care often becomes their primary method of treatment due to the immediate and positive results they get. We also treat patients with other conditions. In theses cases, I use chiropractic adjustments to enhance or support medical treatment by relieving the musculoskeletal aspects associated with their particular condition.

EVALUATING THE PATIENT

I find the most effective method to begin a treatment protocol is to evaluate patients through clinical examination, laboratory testing, diagnostic imaging, and other diagnostic interventions to determine whether chiropractic treatment is right for the patient's condition. Sometimes, I refer patients to the appropriate health care provider when I determine that chiropractic care is not suitable for their condition. Other times, the condition warrants co-management in conjunction with other members of our health care team and we manage all necessary services with in our clinic.

The primary focus of my chiropractic treatment, and any other procedures that we perform in our clinic, is to use the right approach to alleviate the health issue. That's it!

Getting healthier is definitely about lifestyle improvement and the chiropractic adjustment is a powerful tool, but just one of many. The practice of chiropractic manipulative therapy is the most powerful tool that can be applied to physical conditions and does a lot of great things. However, it is not the end all/be all of healthcare. It has to be incorporated and used appropriately when needed, the same way nutrition, rehabilitation, Kinesio® Taping, and anything else must be used to help a patient improve their health and well-being.

PHYSICAL THERAPY IN OUR CLINIC

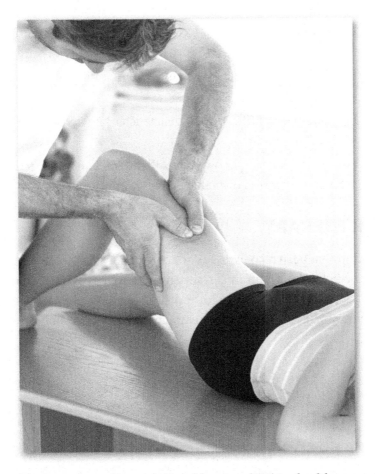

Physical therapy or physiotherapy (often abbreviated PT) is a healthcare profession chiefly concerned with the remediation of impairments and disabilities, and the promotion of mobility, functional ability, quality of life, and movement potential.

Physical therapy utilizes examination, evaluation, diagnosis and physical intervention. Physical therapy can be carried out by a physician (chiropractic or otherwise) or a physical therapist and their assistants. Physical therapy patients have problems or injuries that limit their ability to move and perform functional activities. When applied in the care and well-being of athletes, whether pro, semi-pro, or "weekend warrior", PT usually encompasses complete athletic injury management under 5 main categories:

1. Acute care – working with physician in assessment and diagnosis of an injury;

2. Treatment - application of techniques to encourage healing and painless moving;

3. Rehabilitation - progressive management until able to return to sport;

4. Prevention - identification of deficiencies known to directly result in, or act as precursors to injury

5. Education - sharing knowledge with athletes and their teams to assist in prevention or management of injuries.

LASER THERAPY

Laser therapy has been recognized as one of the many technological therapies that can be helpful for pain in certain areas, as well as skin treatments and cosmetic applications. One application of this new technology with cold laser therapy include pain control treatment for neck and shoulders.

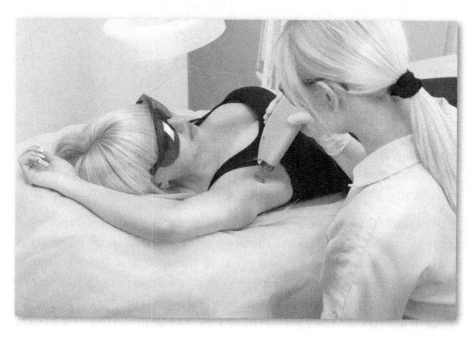

Low level cold lasers have been proven effective in reducing and eliminating acute and chronic pain in the neck & shoulders of patients. Many patients find that laser treatment solution is more effective and a remarkably simple alternative to the use of traditional analgesic pain medications or analgesics with opiates. When Laser therapy is combined with chiropractic adjustments and physical therapy, laser therapy helps patients lead a normal, active, and healthy life without pain.

Cold lasers are currently undergoing studies for use against viruses, scars, burns, wound healing and much more. Although it is a relatively new field of medicine, my commitment to low-level laser treatment has benefitted many patients so far.

FDA Approved

Recently, the FDA created a new regulatory category of medical devices: NHN Biostimulation lasers for the control of cold-laser application devices in healthcare.

MASSAGE THERAPY

Therapeutic Massage involves the use of a state licensed massage therapist to manipulate superficial and deeper muscle layers and connective tissue through various massage techniques that tend to enhance function, aid in natural healing, decrease muscle reflex reactions, promote relaxation, and improve health.

In a therapeutic massage, the patient is massaged while lying on a special table built for massage therapy, or while sitting on chair especially designed for massage. The patient may be fully or partially clothed.

If you are injured, massage therapy plays a vital role in your healing process. Massage involves working with acting on muscles, tendons, ligaments, fascia, skin, joints or connective tissue. Areas targeted by the massage therapist, under the guidance of your doctor, might include hands, fingers, elbows, knees, forearm, or feet, as well as the cervical, thoracic, or lumbar spine as well as your stomach.

Massage can also assist in the proper drainage of the lymphatic system. Proper drainage is critical for the elimination of waste products from the body. Massage therapy promotes this elimination process while mobilizing soft tissue at the same time.

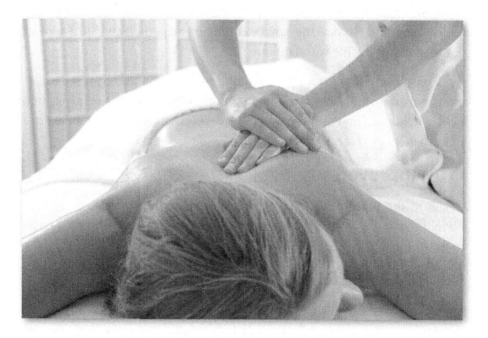

Massage Therapy provides great benefit for the following conditions:

- Muscle spasms, tension, and stiffness
- Limited ROM (range of motion) of the muscles and joints
- Restricted circulation of blood and movement of lymph flows
- Promotion of faster healing of soft tissue injuries
- Reduction of scar tissue
- Improvement in posture
- Reduction in overall stress and anxiety, thus creating a feeling of well-being
- Promotion of a relaxed state of mental awareness

FUNCTIONAL EXERCISE

The term "function" as it's applied in functional exercise, training, rehabilitation and testing is really used to describe work aimed at helping athletes reach their movement goals. Functional Exercise creates restoration of strength and agility through dynamic movement in Functional Rehabilitation.

During Functional Exercise, several muscle groups are exercised simultaneously. A set of exercises is usually sport-specific, and typically specialized equipment is required. It's sufficient to say that our approach is in many ways more practical, appropriate, efficient and holistic. We discuss functional exercise in greater detail in the Neuro-Stabilization chapter of this book.

KINESIO® TAPING

You've seen it used with professional football players and Olympic athletes, so what is it?

Kinesio® Taping gives strength and stability to your joints and muscles without affecting circulation and range of motion. It is also used for preventive maintenance, edema, and to treat pain.

We use Kinesio® tape quite uniquely and perhaps not entirely as intended, but it works great. We use Kinesio® tape to stimulate muscle spindles and golgi tendons to promote and inhibit muscular function. I call it the Neuro-tape.

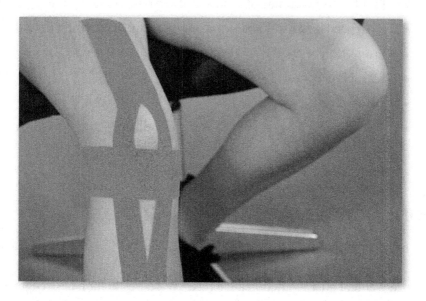

Kinesio® Taping is a technique based on the body's own natural healing process. This Kinesio® Taping exhibits its efficiency through the activation of neurological and circulatory systems. The method stems from the science of Kinesiology (*def.: the study of the principles of mechanics and anatomy in relation to human movement*), hence the name "Kinesio."

Muscles are not only responsible for body movements but also control the circulation of venous and lymph flows, body temperature, etc. Therefore, if the muscles don't function properly, it causes a myriad of symptoms. Kinesio® Taping creates a totally different treatment approach for nerves, muscles and organs.

The first documented use of Kinesio® Taping was for a patient with articular disorders. For the first 10 years, orthopedists, chiropractors, acupuncturists and other medical practitioners were the primary users of Kinesio® Taping. Kinesio® Taping was used by the Japanese Olympic volleyball team and word quickly spread to other athletes. Today, Kinesio® Taping is used by medical practitioners and athletes around the world.

Kinesio® Tape is used for anything from headaches to foot problems and everything in between. Examples include: muscular facilitation or inhibition in pediatric patients, carpal tunnel syndrome treatment, alleviation of lower back strain/pain (subluxations, herniated discs). It's also highly effective in treating knee conditions, shoulder conditions, hamstring, groin injury, rotator cuff injury, whiplash, tennis elbow, plantar fasciitis, patella tracking, pre- and post-surgical edema, ankle sprains and athletic preventative injury method, and is also used as a support method.

Conventional athletic tape was originally designed to restrict the movement of affected muscles and joints. For this purpose, several layers of tape were rolled around and/or over the afflicted area, while applying significant pressure, resulting in the obstruction of the flow of bodily fluids as an undesirable side-effect.

This is also the reason.Kinesio® athletic tape is usually applied immediately before the sports activity, and removed immediately after the activity is finished. Kinesio® Taping is NOT a supportive tape job, so the tape is highly flexible. It doesn't prevent movement; it allows the muscles to go through their full range of motion.

It also allows the joints to bend and move, so it's not supportive like an athletic training taping job. Kinesio® Taping is a neurologic taping technique that allows the muscles to function and over a course of one to three days, depending on how long the tape adheres, it helps train the human mind to understand what the body needs to do, and how it should be doing it.

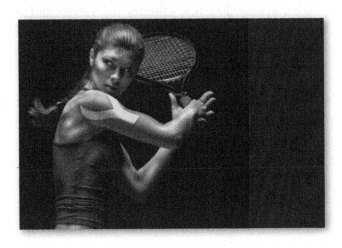

ELECTRICAL MUSCLE STIMULATION

Electrical muscle stimulation, or EMS therapy, is used to treat a variety of painful issues, much like therapeutic massage, from muscle strain and injury to fibromyalgia symptoms.

EMS is a commonly sought-after treatment that uses an electrotherapy device that delivers a small, pulsating current to the muscles and nerve endings. This current encourages blood circulation, muscle stimulation and healing.

One of the greater benefits of Electrical Muscle Stimulation (EMS) is that it can be used as therapy to treat weak or atrophied muscles resulting from an injury or from long periods of immobility. This works by stimulating muscles, which causes them to contract and relax, much like normal physical activity. The Electrical Muscular Stimulation helps develop strength in the affected area and can be used to treat completely incapacitated patients because EMS therapeutic treatment creates involuntary muscle contraction responses, thereby improving and also maintaining muscle tone without any actual physical activity.

Many sports-related injuries reduce the range of motion in joints, especially in the shoulders, elbows and knees. EMS can be used on an impeded joint to increase range of motion and promote healing in the injured area by increasing blood flood and thereby reducing inflammation.

Many of my patients suggest that EMS helps relieve their chronic pain in joints and muscles, as well as their suffering from stress and tension. EMS is great for relieving pain in patients with fibromyalgia and also can be used to treat chronic headaches, muscle weakness and fatigue, as well as overall body aches and pain.

Because of the restricted range of motion in tender and swollen joints, EMS therapy works well for arthritis sufferers by increasing range of motion in their joints and reducing pain and inflammation. EMS does this by channeling a low-frequency electrical current through muscle nerves and the connective tissue. Pain relief is accomplished when the body begins secreting additional amounts of endorphins and other natural pain relievers to the affected area.

HOW EMS WORKS

Electrical Muscular Stimulation works by placing electrodes at the site of the injury and gradually increasing the electrical current output. What the patient feels in the beginning is a tingling sensation. As the electrical current increases, the tingling feels stronger but not uncomfortable in any way. Over a short period of time, the patient's body adapts to the electrical current, which necessitates an increase in the electrical current level every few minutes. A typical EMS treatment lasts from 10 to 20 minutes, depending on the condition being treated.

Some of the more common injuries that are treated with EMS include strained ligaments, muscle sprains, strains and spasms.

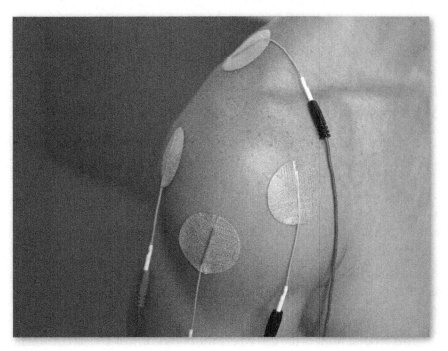

MICROCURRENT THERAPY

Microcurrent therapy, commonly referred as MENS (Microcurrent Electrical Neuromuscular Stimulation), is similar to EMS therapy, yet differs in that MENS uses an extremely tiny pulsating electrical current.

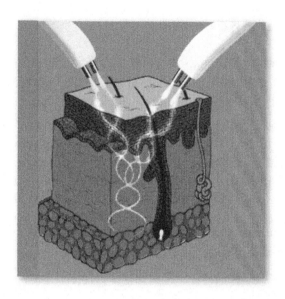

These microcurrents are finely tuned to the level of the normal electrical exchanges that occur at the body's cellular level, as opposed to the EMS which deals with stimulating nerve endings, muscles and ligaments. The micro currents penetrate into the cell, contrary to passing over it as EMS does.

Microcurrent therapy works on something called the Ardnt-Schultz Law, which states: *"Weak stimuli increase physiological activity and very strong stimuli will inhibit or abolish physiological activity."*

This microcurrent therapy helps balance the activity taking place within the cell if the cell had been injured or otherwise compromised. The external addition of micro currents increases the production of ATP, protein synthesis, oxygenation, ion exchange, absorption of nutrients, elimination of waste products, and neutralizes the oscillating polarity of deficient cells. Balance is thereby restored.

This process bridges the gap where the body's own electrical current fails, as the human body must adhere to the natural law of electricity, which is: *"electricity must take the path of least resistance."* The theory is that an electric current tends to move around an injury or defect, rather than through it.

The MENS normalizes cell activity, and therefore, reduces inflammation while increasing collagen-producing cells. The MENS therapy assists the body in creating the perfect environment for self-healing. It helps stimulate an electrical field at the cellular level to improve circulation, and helps the blood flow more actively through the affected area. It uses more oxygen and promotes an accelerated and more natural healing.

ULTRASOUND

You may think of it as the technology used to see unborn fetuses, but Ultrasound has great applications. Ultrasound Therapy (US) is done with a wand device that creates sound waves (outside of our range of hearing) and directs them into your body. An ultrasound device can be used to treat injuries.

The sound waves produced by an Ultrasound machine can penetrate up to 4 inches deep from skin level. At that depth the sound waves are absorbed and produce a heat sensation. (You might compare this to a hot pack on the outside of your body, but the hot pack only penetrates inches in.) Sound waves also tend to stimulate things a bit. Let me give you an analogy. Imagine putting a tablespoon of salt into water. It will dissolve by itself, but if you stir it with the spoon, it dissolves immediately. That's a good comparison for the effect that Ultrasound vibrations have on accelerating your body's own natural healing abilities.

Ultrasound therapy can relax muscles, tendons, ligaments, increase blood flow and has been used to break down scar tissue. Ultrasound is absorbed by soft tissue such as ligaments, muscles, fascia and scar tissue which makes it a valid and sought after therapy for sprains, and strains, plus acute chronic issues.

Typically Ultrasound therapy sessions will be 3-5 minutes in length, depending on how big an area the treatment is needed for. Treatment to break down scar tissue takes a bit longer. You will not feel anything during Ultrasound other than the wand sensation as it is touching you.

Case study .....Injury Care:

Because of my background, I tend to see the bigger, stronger people walking through my door. At 42 Years of age, a power lifter presented with radiating pain into his right arm and weakness and numbness in the right hand. He was concerned because he was showing obvious weakness in the right arm and hand in comparison to the left. He had seen his orthopedic surgeon who first suggested a shot and 4 weeks of physical therapy. After 4 weeks of physical therapy, he felt no improvement and indicated that the weakness was worsening. His second visit to the orthopedist was an immediate suggestion to do surgery on the neck. He was told that was the only option left.

After a comprehensive orthopedic/neurologic exam and review of the X-rays and MRI, we determined that his issue originated in his neck. He had an issue called thoracic outlet syndrome that was causing the numbness in the arm as well as a neck issue that was radiating pain.

This patient was treated with a total of 8 visits over a 4 week period of time. He was treated with chiropractic manipulative therapies, very basic rehabilitation exercises targeted for TOS (Thoracic Outlet Syndrome is a group of disorders that occur when the blood vessels or nerves in the space between your collarbone and your first rib, the thoracic outlet, become compressed), and Kinesio® Taping was utilized to reset muscle spindles, turning down muscles that were too tight and getting the muscles that were not working properly functioning again. At the end of week 4, this patient no longer presented with any signs of weakness or any symptoms of pain or numbness.

This gentleman is now a friend of mine and 3 months after his treatment ended he placed 3rd in a national power-lifting meet.

Chapter 4

Neuro-Stabilization Training

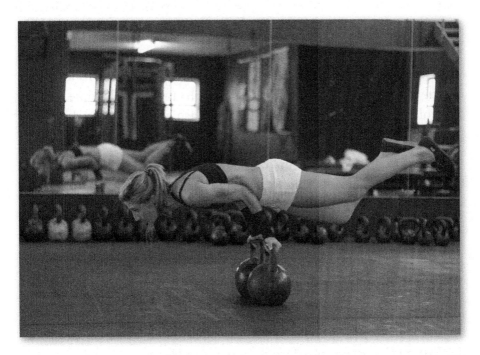

Neuro-Stabilization Training creates an energy-efficient, stable, strong, flexible, and dynamically useful Neuro-Musculoskeletal System. Neuro-Stabilization training involves and incorporates the body's ability to create stability around joints, while training the central nervous system to coordinate muscular control in a more efficient and effective way. Neuro-stabilization training involves a thought process with endless possibilities. The question that you have to keep asking is "How could I make this movement harder or create more instability

while continuing to perform it correctly?" Because this question is not specific, it can be applied to any action, drill, exercise, etc.

Neuro-Stabilization Training can also be applied to and enhance any other form of training (power training, speed training, cross-fit, TRX, kettle bell, etc.) Neuro-Stabilization Training helps reduce the risk of injury by creating stability and, in turn, building your strength.

There are endless options for increasing the difficulty of the exercises and therefore limitless potential for improving athletic performance and making your body stronger. One of the greatest benefits of Neuro-Stabilization Training is that it increases your stabilization capacity and can be adapted for any sport-specific training.

Your brain is aware of more than your movement patterns and your muscle groups: your brain understands stabilization. While some athletes are isolating muscle groups for training, wise athletes are looking into Neuro- Stabilization Training.

To start with, you must follow simple patterns of movement and pay close attention to how they occur, one after the other (in the developmental sequence beginning when you are born) and developing throughout your childhood and into adolescence.

Your most essential activities revolve around simple movements of running and climbing. When you are running, your body requires that you have a stable spine and that you are able to transfer power from one leg to the other also your body must deal with the movement of the arms (counterbalance) as they swing. On the other hand, when climbing, you need your spine to be more flexible and adaptable.

Once you start working on Neuro-stabilization, core strengthening can be accomplished through functional movements.

The Mitchell Principle

The "Mitchell Principle" is *the proper performance of an activity while placed upon a dynamically unstable surface, increasing the dynamic stability of the joints and joint stabilizers. It increases proprioception and strength while reducing the risk of injury, and it increases the body's ability to perform that action.*

This criterion is used to prepare the nervous system resulting in enhanced coordination and motor control while placing the athlete in an increasingly greater proprioceptive-rich environment. Proprioception will be discussed in detail later in this chapter.

I'm obviously a firm believer in developing stability training. I'm a Power-Lifter and I depend on stabilization.

You can't be strong until you're stable. Have you ever tried to push something away from you when you were treading water? (Picture trying to push a shark away while you are treading water. Got it?)

(It's not too easy to create strength, power, and force in this scenario.)

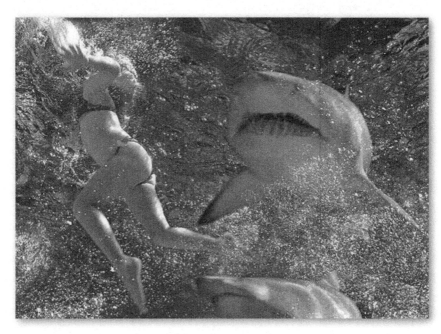

You must have core stability and joint stability, and for that to occur, you have to train properly for it. One way to accomplish this is to conduct your training on an unstable surface, like the Bosu ball. When you perform an activity on a dynamically unstable surface all of your stabilizing muscles must stabilize the joint, and it is the prime movers that actually move the ball, the weight or whatever is being moved.

Building core muscles and core stability are critically essential in preventing injuries. It is equally vital to create joint stability (stability of the auxiliary muscles that surround each joint). The only way to create true joint stability is to push the athlete to stabilize within the activity (or movement) that they're performing, whatever it may be: pitching a fastball, kicking a soccer ball to goal, leaping to the top of a cheerleading squad pyramid or throwing a football.

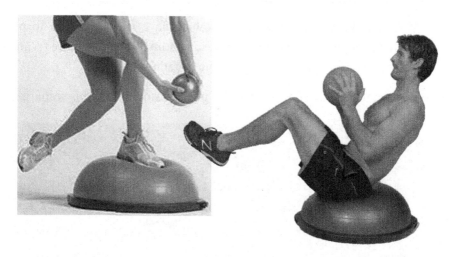

Specialized equipment that we employ to increase core and joint stability is also available to our patients to use at home. One such piece of equipment is called a Bosu ball, shown above.

One side of the Bosu ball is a flat board, and the other side is an inflated ball. A Bosu ball can help athletes take simple exercises to the next level, creating core and joint stability specifically for those special motions they use the most. For instance, all of the following can be done using the Bosu ball (variations: kneeling on a stability ball):

- Throwing a pitch (use two Bosu balls: with one foot on the Bosu, step to the next Bosu, and then throw a pitch.)
- Swinging a golf club
- Catching a football
- Shooting a basketball

When these athletic activities are performed on an unstable surface, they tend to build great core stability as well as joint stability, and those are the key factors in preventing injuries and/or tissue damage, even for athletes functioning at an exceptionally high level of performance.

PROPRIOCEPTION - Proprioception: Heard of it before today? Probably not!

We have five common senses that we learn about from an early age: sight, hearing, taste, touch and smell. Our consciousness is very aware of the function of these senses. The conscious part of the brain has complete awareness of those 5 senses. Our conscious awareness voluntarily checks up on data received from these 5 senses as they experience their surroundings, and typically, when a sufficient stimuli has brought conscious attention to those sensors.

One overlooked sense, called proprioception, is vitally important for normal functioning. "Proprioception is the way that the body can vary its muscle contractions in immediate response to the data it receives regarding incoming information about the external environment." It does this by using stretch abilities, or stretch receptor in our muscles to track the joint position.

You might think of it like balance, but it's really far more complex than balance. You see, literally every joint in the body must communicate to the brain what position it is in before you can begin moving. How can you bend your arm if you don't know that it is straight, but not only is it straight, but how straight it is?

Let's give you a little example that's easy to understand. What happens when you step on the pointy end of a tack (barefoot of course)? Your reflexes will usually remove your foot from the tack immediately and remove the tack. We all do that! That reaction by our body is so fast that the feeling of stepping on that tack doesn't even get relayed to our brain before we pull our foot off of the tack. This is a reflex action, called a reaction, that relays information back to the spinal cord and then back out to the foot at an unreal rate of speed.

So, if the pain signal doesn't move to our brain, how do we know to move our foot away from danger and/or not to fall over? The answer is - proprioception. Proprioception is so important that it runs on the fastest and largest track of our nervous system to get information to our brain instantaneously. The proprioceptive input to our brain, in this scenario, is that the position that our body is in at the time of the tack-stepping episode gets relayed, processed and integrated into our brain faster than the time it took for the pain to return to the spinal cord. That's fast!

PROPRIOCEPTION AND ATHLETIC PERFORMANCE

THE NERVOUS SYSTEM:

Some people just seem more athletically gifted. Everyone knows 'those' people that just have it and 'those others' that don't. If you have read Malcolm Gladwell's book "Outliers", you might say that this does not matter when becoming an exceptionally high level performer in your sport.

In Gladwell's book, the Principle of 10,000 hours of practice is discussed in detail. He relates this to not only sports performance, but to all aspects of life and the people that are truly "Outliers". This principle has a lot of merit, and that is because of our Central Nervous System.

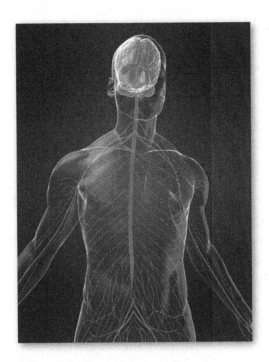

THE CENTRAL NERVOUS SYSTEM

The central nervous system runs from your brain to the tail of your spinal cord. This structure of your body coordinates and controls every aspect of how your body functions. Walking, talking, chewing gum, breathing, thinking, circulating blood and everything else is coordinated and controlled by the central nervous system (CNS).

If your body was a computer, then the CNS is the CPU or central processing unit, and the other structures of our bodies are the monitors, video card, RAM memory, mouse, keyboard, etc... None of the other structures of our bodies will work without input from the CNS.

The greatest aspect of our CNS is that it is remarkably plastic. Plasticity means pliable, malleable or changeable. The Central Nervous System has the ability to adapt and reconfigure itself to make things happen the way you want them to work, and what this actually means is that it can be trained to do just about anything. This, in turn, means our bodies can be trained to do just about anything as well.

The plasticity or versatility of the brain might be better explained if I described a case I had not long ago. She, unfortunately, had brain cancer and had undergone multiple surgeries resulting in the removal of nearly 1/3 of the right side of her brain. Within 6 to 9 months the opposite side of her brain took over the role of the surgically removed part. This patient was over 50 years of age so just think about what a younger, developing brain can do!

THE PERIPHERAL NERVOUS SYSTEM

The lines of communication to the other structures in our bodies are known as the Peripheral Nervous System (PNS). Again, if our body were a computer, the CNS would be your central processing unit, and the PNS would be the cords to the monitor, mouse, keyboard, etc. Imagine the wiring diagram of a highly sophistical technological device.

The PNS comes off of the spinal cord as nerve roots. These roots then proceed to branch off, time and time again, until they reach the end cells of our body. We have trillions of cells and the PNS has to get to them all, so each nerve root controls billions of cells. All of the data to and from each end cell gets relayed back first to the spinal cord, then up to the brain, and is integrated by the brain, back down the spinal cord, and finally back out to that end cell.

This sounds like a complicated process because it is, but if you think of it as a computer, it makes it much easier to understand.

THE CEREBELLUM

The cerebellum is a smaller part of the CNS that integrates and coordinates the precision and accuracy of your movements. It is the controlling aspect of how coordinated you are as an athlete or non-athlete.

Are you someone that seems to be "accident prone" or "falls down frequently"? This tendency is primarily based on cerebellar activity. In athletics, the physical coordination to kick a soccer ball, throw a baseball, catch a football, comes down to the neural integration of movement by the cerebellum.

How accurate or inaccurate you are in these activities is based upon how well the cerebellum is trained or functioning.

MUSCLES DON'T HAVE MEMORY!

Training of the cerebellum would be considered motor learning, which to most of us means practicing the skill correctly, over and over again. The learning and memory processes do not come from the muscle at all. The muscles and the coordination of neuron firing patterns that go into performing a skill come from motor learning in the cerebellum. However, before the cerebellum can synchronize any motor movement, it must first know where the body is in space and against gravity. This is a part of proprioception that we mentioned earlier.

PROPRIOCEPTION EXAMPLE

Let's try this. Stand and balance on one foot. Make sure your legs are not touching one another. Now close your eyes while remaining in this position; you will realize this task is not so easy. You'll discover that it will be much harder for you to stay balanced when you close your eyes. This is because your balance is primarily determined by 3 mechanisms in your body, and with your eyes closed you lose your perception of where you are in space. The 2 of the 3 determining mechanisms of balance are:

The vestibular system: This system is located in the inner ear and helps to coordinate balance and spatial orientation. The vestibular system sends signals to the brain to coordinate eye movements and to muscle to keep us standing upright.

Vision: When your eyes are open, your brain is constantly working to keep your eyes level with the horizon, which helps keep you balanced.

And the third mechanism of balance is...

PROPRIOCEPTION

In this example, there is a bone in your ankle called the talus. This bone has no muscular attachments, which means that it is not moved by muscles like almost all other bones are. Instead, this bone creates a joint complex in the ankle that has a large volume of proprioceptive input to the brain. The bone is almost like a little gyroscope in the ankle, constantly sending proprioceptive signals to the brain, telling your brain what position you are in.

When you close your eyes, you have just removed one of the three mechanisms, vision. Now your body is forced to rely on the vestibular system and the quality of proprioceptive input from the ankle. What you'll notice is that your foot becomes "unquiet" or unsteady immediately. This makes maintaining your balance much harder.

THE CEREBELLUM, PROPRIOCEPTION and ATHLETIC PERFORMANCE

Athleticism (the ability for a person to engage in athletics) is for the most part based on proprioception and cerebellum activity. So, our athletic ability rests solely on the function of our nervous system, which has a vast amount of plasticity and can be trained.

The training process involves learning to coordinate your movement in ways that are effective and beneficial uses of our energy. The more you prepare yourself to coordinate motor patterns in energy efficient ways, the easier it is for you to perform the activity. The easier it gets to perform that activity, the faster and better you can accomplish that activity.

If you can perform an action better or faster than your competitor, then you are better than them and you have a higher probability of winning. Simply put, the better your nervous system functions the better you perform as an athlete during your sports activity, or as an everyday person in your everyday life. This is what Neuro-Stabilization training is all about.

CORE STRENGTHENING / TRAINING

Core stability is the ability to transfer energy to the extremities without energy insufficiencies that decrease joint stability. There are two types of core strengthening: Voluntary and Involuntary.

Voluntary core strengthening involves the deliberate contraction of the core in an isolated movement. There are three methods of voluntary core training. The first two methods were developed by Richardson, Hodges, and Jull, and this was covered in their book: *Therapeutic Exercise for Spinal Segmental Stabilization in Low Back Pain*. The first method is called - drawing in. In this method, you suck your belly button in toward your spine. The second method is the hollowing method, which is remarkably similar to drawing in, although it should reduce the waist diameter if done correctly. The third method is bracing, which was developed by Stuart McGill in his books *Low Back Disorders & Ultimate Back Fitness and Performance*. This method is a simultaneous co-activation of the transverse abdominus, internal obliques, external obliques, and rectus abdominus.

Involuntary Core Strengthening involves the involuntary contraction of the core musculature to stabilize the performed movement. Involuntary core contraction and strengthening happens when the person is forced to stabilize the body before performing an action. This is achieved by performing that action on a dynamically unstable surface.

This is the core training routine I use for myself, and it incorporates Neuro-Stabilization movements far better than the voluntary contraction work. That is not to say that the voluntary contraction of the core is not beneficial, but consistent voluntary contraction of the core is impractical in everyday life.

Specific core training needs to be done in conjunction with the forced involuntary core contraction exercises. There are hundreds if not thousands of core specific exercises that strengthen the individual/athlete.

TECHNIQUE IS EVERYTHING

When it comes to Neuro-Stabilization Training, technique is everything. The better the technique, the more efficient you are with your movements, the easier, smoother and safer those movements become. Dynamically unstable surfaces make for better technique. Think about it like this: have you ever seen someone breaking their backs while lifting something off the ground? If they were standing on an unstable surface, they would fall flat on their face. The unstable surface makes your body fire stabilizing muscles before you start lifting and puts you in proper posture, or you can't lift whatever it is.

The Basics Principles of Neuro-Stabilization Training:

1. Any exercise that can be performed while standing can be performed while standing on a dynamically unstable surface.

2. Any exercise that can be done while lying on a bench can be performed lying over a stability ball.

3. Properly performing activities without a counter balance increases the body's ability to stabilize itself.

4. The greater the dynamically unstable environment is when the activity is properly performed, the greater the dynamic stability of the body during that activity.

BEFORE YOU PERFORM

You would think by now there would be concrete data, evidence, or at least an cross-the-board industry standard about how to prepare the body for activity, but there isn't. Everyone seems to have their own approach and thoughts on the matter. This would be my approach:

• Foam Roll

• Light Generalized Dynamic Warm-up Exercises

• Static & Dynamic Stretching

• Dynamic Warm-ups, within the activity to be performed.

FOAM ROLLING

Foam rolling muscle essentially softens the muscles and makes them more pliable. Pliability of muscle is beneficial when used in a dynamic fashion. Playing a sport or training is using muscle in a dynamic fashion. When muscles are injured or overworked, they tend to become fibrotic. The fascial tissue contracts around the muscle, increasing the density of the muscle.

Foam rolling works well to break this fascial tissue down and soften the muscle itself.

DYNAMIC GENERALIZED WARM UP

Warm-up is extremely crucial. This kind of warm up would be non-sport/ activity specific. Basic general dynamic are those exercises that loosen up the entire body, increase overall blood circulation and lymphatic drainage and increase respiration. Examples of such exercises, include but are not limited to:

- High Knee Walking
- Leg Swings Squats: Lateral and Vertical
- Lunges
- Chin Tucks with Scapular Tightening
- Calf Raises and Toe Raises
- Wall Angels

STRETCHING:

Don't cut corners. Be sure to stretch. The purpose of stretching is to literally lengthen the muscle. Chronically shortened muscles don't have the same amount of contractile force and don't perform as well as muscles that are lengthened and provide full range of motion to joints. Stretching is performed after the muscles have been significantly warmed-up. Stretching should be a combination of static and dynamic activities.

Stretching in general helps to minimize injury, increases joint range of motion, creates flexibility in the muscles and increases muscular performance. Remember that your body has to be properly hydrated (at least 2 liters of purified water a day) to be flexible.

SPORTS/ACTIVITY SPECIFIC WARM-UP:

Don't jump from stretching to sprinting. Warm-up in the activity you are about to perform and take the time to do it properly and thoroughly. This allows your nervous system to adjust the muscles' firing patterns for the activity. This also allows your body to increase blood flow to the area in demand.

Cold muscles don't perform well and must be warmed up with increased blood circulation. With increased blood flow, comes the necessary nutrients and oxygen needed for performance. Cold muscles are less pliable and at high risk of injury. To maximize prevention and performance, warm up your muscles!

Case Study:

At 52 years of age, a weight trainer presented with right shoulder pain. He indicated that the pain increased when he tried to use the shoulder and that he had not been able to weight train for over a month due to pain. He rated his shoulder pain at a level of 8/10 when he tried to use it in the gym. I was the initial physician to see him for this injury.

After examining him, I determined that he appeared to have an impingement issue with his supraspinatus tendon. This would be considered rotator cuff syndrome.

We started a treatment plan that included modified weight training once we had the inflammation of the shoulder under control. We implemented Neuro-Stabilization training to his weight training regimen and within 6 weeks he was as "strong as he has ever been", in multiple lifts, however he continued to have dull 1/10 pain with certain activities. I then ordered an MRI to rule out anything that was non-musculoskeletal. What came back was extremely surprising. He had a full thickness tear of his supraspinatous muscle. How we were able to get him back to what he was doing with minimal to no pain was unbelievable. Unfortunately, I needed to send him to an orthopedic surgeon to have the tear repaired. Afterward, we provided his post- surgical rehabilitation and he is now pain free and continuing to perform all activities without restrictions.

Chapter 5

Concussions/Traumatic Brain Injuries

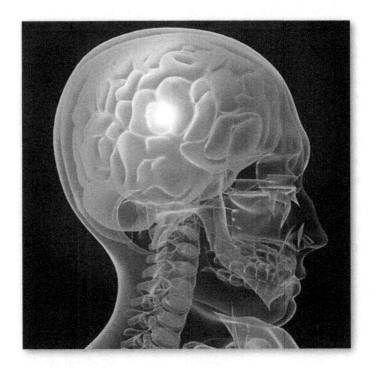

DESCRIPTION OF A CONCUSSION

Concussions can be and are life-altering experiences. It is absolutely essential that players, coaches and people in general, become more educated about what concussions are, how to help prevent them and their proper treatment.

Prevention and treatment of concussions is so crucial that I've written an entire chapter about it. Through learning about concussions, their treatment and how to prevent them you'll also discover ways to improve your athletic performance by improving your functional, neurologic mechanisms.

The Mayo clinic defines a concussion as:

"A traumatic brain injury that alters the way your brain functions. Effects are usually temporary, but can include problems with headache, concentration, memory, judgment, balance and coordination."

That means that if you do get a concussion, the condition is usually temporary, but can be life altering for years afterward if not treated correctly. You can most likely improve your situation with functional neurologic exercises.

Though usually caused by a blow to the head, concussions can also occur when the head and upper body are violently shaken. If left untreated, the injured person can continue to concuss physiologically (chemically) without any further trauma to the head. Concussive injuries can cause loss of consciousness, but not usually. Because of this some people experience a concussion and don't even realize that it has occurred.

Marshall, et al, Sports related concussions: JCCA 2012; "Concussion is due to abrupt linear and or rotational acceleration or deceleration of the brain within the skull."

Here are some compelling statistics concerning concussions:

- For females, playing soccer accounts for the most concussions, and for males, gridiron football accounts for nearly 50% of all concussions.

- 1.7 million people (including 475,000 children) sustain traumatic brain injuries per year in the US.

- 3.1 million individuals live with life-long disabilities as the result of their injuries.

- Traumatic brain injuries account for 30% of all injury related deaths in the US.

- Seventy-five percent of traumatic brain injuries are concussions.

Source: www.biausa.org : Brain Injury Association of America

DANGERS OF CONCUSSIONS

Recent evidence indicates that repeated concussions cause cumulative brain damage, and the damage shows up as chronic neuropsychological deficits which tend to result in social dysfunction, lost productivity time, and excessive healthcare costs (B W Benson et al. British Journal of Sports Medicine 2002).

Concussions are vastly underestimated in the sports world. I personally feel that there needs to be an environment created where the patient/athlete is treated properly, not just sent home to rest with sunglasses, pain killers, and an ice bag on their head, and without proper follow-up.

Considering the growing incidents of concussions resulting from sports, it appears that there aren't sufficient healthcare practitioners who actually treat concussions for neuro-functional control. Very few practitioners are doing anything to stimulate the areas of the brain that have been concussed in order for the injured person's brain to recover more quickly with reduced long-term adverse, or life-threatening effects.

Treating concussions is a specialty in the field of sports medicine and it is one of the specialties at our clinic as well. Our approach is an integrative one, with physicians who initially treat the injury and later provide the aftercare needed for thorough healing. In my opinion, this is the best approach for treatment of concussions.

There are many causes of a concussion, causes that are greatly increased especially when you are involved with sports or if you are extraordinarily active. It is just so rare that a concussion is treated with little more than films, pain medication, sunglasses, and ice packs.

Recently, sports-related concussions have become a really hot topic, because there is a lot of media exposure regarding pro athletes who have suffered from repeated concussions, and exhibit the many debilitating effects of long-term damage that can happen with repeated concussions. To date, medical science doesn't really comprehend the full impact and long-term effects of having multiple contusions.

"In my clinic, I am regularly treating an increasing number of high school athletes with concussions."

According to researchers (Theye, et al. "Heads Up": Concussions I High School Sports - a review, Clinical Medicine and Research. 2004.) high school athletes are more susceptible to concussions, and they take longer to heal. High school athletes seem to recover about one week slower than their college-age counterparts. These younger athletes are also about three times more likely to have a second concussion in the same season as the first one. We call this "Second Impact Syndrome" and it can be caused by trauma, as well as the chemical after-effects of the first concussion, as I mentioned earlier.

My strongest belief is that it is vital that athletes are properly evaluated immediately after the concussion, just as they would be for any other injury that requires emergency care.

Table 1
– Signs and Symptoms of Concussion from the American College of Sports Medicine updated consensus statement – 2011[1]. Reprinted with permission from Herring SA, Cantu RC, Guskiewicz KM, Putukian M, Kibler WB, Bergfeld JA, et al. Concussion (mild traumatic brain injury) and the team physician: a consensus statement – 2011 update. Medicine & Science in Sports & Exercise. 2011; 2412–22.

Cognitive	Somatic	Affective	Sleep Disturbance
– Confusion – Amnesia (Retrograde or Anterograde) – Loss of Consciousness – Disorientation – Feeling "in a fog", or "zoned out" – Vacant stare – Inability to focus – Delayed verbal and motor responses – Slurred/incoherent speech – Excessive drowsiness	– Headache – Dizziness – Balance Disruption – Nausea/Vomiting – Visual Disturbances – Phonophobia	– Emotional Lability – Irritability – Fatigue – Anxiety – Sadness	– Trouble falling asleep – Sleeping more than usual – Sleeping less than usual

Table 4

Return to play stages as outlined by the 3rd International Conference on Concussion in Sport, held in Zurich in 2008.[2]
*Each of these stages is to take at least 24 hours. If any symptoms are incurred at any one of the stages, the athlete is to
take the rest of the day off and return to the previous stage the following day. The athlete is to remain at that stage for
at least 24 hours. If symptom free, they may attempt the next stage again.*

Graduated Return to Play Protocol		
Stage of Rehab	**Functional Exercise to be attempted**	**Objectives to meet**
1. No Activity	Complete physical and cognitive rest	Recovery – remain at stage 1 until symptom free
2. Light aerobic exercise*	Walking, swimming, stationary cycling (Intensity <70% of max heart (HR) rate) – no resistance training	Increase HR
3. Sport-specific exercise	Skating, running, jumping (No head impact activities)	Add sport-specific movement
4. Non-contact training drills	Progress to more complex training drills (passing, catching, dribbling, stick-handling etc.); May begin progressive resistance training	Exercise, coordination, and cognitive load – challenging multiple systems
5. Full contact practice**	Following medical clearance, participate in normal training activities	Restore confidence and assess functional skills
6. Return to play	Normal Game Play	

* - Prior to returning to exercise, the authors recommend adding in a cognitive stage in which the athlete attempts a period of
    reading and light cognitive activities
** - Prior to returning the athlete to full contact, ensure that he or she has been sufficiently challenged cognitively and physically
     with high intensity exercise and complex training drills

SIGNS AND SYMPTOMS

While we glossed-over some of the symptoms above, concussions are something that just can't be ignored. A more in depth examination is needed to learn how to diagnose and treat what can be a particularly serious even life-threatening injury. According to the Mayo Clinic, the signs and symptoms of a concussion can be subtle and may not be immediately apparent. Symptoms can last for days, weeks, or even longer.

One very serious concern that people often miss about concussions is that the onset of symptoms may be delayed by hours or days after the initial injury.

According to the Mayo Clinic, people may experience the following symptoms with a delayed onset:

- Concentration and memory complaints
- Irritability and other personality changes
- Sensitivity to light and noise
- Sleep disturbances
- Psychological adjustment issues and depression
- Taste and smell disorders

CHILDREN AND CONCUSSIONS

More research has been done on children and concussions since concussions with children are fairly commonplace. As I have stated earlier, they should be treated within the appropriate time frames. It is sometimes difficult to diagnose a young child with a concussion, but you can look for these symptoms:

- Listlessness, tiring easily
- Irritability, crankiness
- Change in eating or sleeping patterns
- Lack of interest in favorite toys
- Loss of balance, unsteady walking

The American Academy of Pediatrics recommends that you call your child's doctor for advice if your child receives anything more than a light bump on the head. If your child remains alert, moves normally, and responds to you, the injury is probably minimal and usually doesn't need further testing. In this case, if your child wants to nap, it's OK to let them sleep.

If worrisome signs develop later, seek emergency care. I would take this one step further because even a mild concussion should be evaluated for further treatment. Injuries in young athletes can be cumulative if not treated promptly, or if they return to play too early.

According to the Mayo Clinic staff, you should not wait for emergency care if you or someone you are caring for has a head injury and begins experiencing the following symptoms:

- Vomiting
- Headache that worsens over time
- Changes in his or her behavior, including irritability or fussiness
- Changes in physical coordination, including stumbling or clumsiness
- Confusion or disorientation

- Slurred speech or other changes in speech
- Vision or eye disturbances, including pupils that are bigger than normal (dilated pupils) or pupils of varying sizes
- Changes in breathing pattern
- Lasting or recurrent dizziness
- Blood or fluid discharge from the nose or ears
- Large head bumps or bruises on areas other than the forehead, especially in infants under 12 months of age

TRUE-BASELINE ATHLETIC ASSESSMENT

In our clinic we have created a baseline assessment of athletes that gives us a more accurate read on any underlying issues that may need to be addressed with the athlete.

The current concussion baseline test is typically a computerized test that quite frankly is NOT enough. It is easy to do, however it only incorporates cognitive function of the brain. The brain controls so much more than the ability to reason, and the test has inherent flaws such as: is the athlete tanking the test on purpose so they would be able to play even after a head injury occurred. Does the child have current deficits due to previous head trauma that now becomes their baseline function? Does the child have proprioceptive or cerebellar issues which would present with balance testing as opposed to cognitive reasoning, etc... The list goes on and on.

This doesn't make the computer testing bad; in fact, it is a great tool, just not the only tool that should be used when making assessments on brain injuries or concussions.

OUR TRUE-BASELINE ATHLETIC ASSESSMENT

- True-Baseline Athletic Assessment. the purpose of the entire assessment is to establish a baseline on all of the characteristics that we would see an athlete for medically. That is to say, if something does occur we a have comparative analysis to reference for severity of the injury. Also, it allows undetected functional deficiencies to be discovered before it leads to an injury. These deficiencies can be rehabbed during the off-season strength and conditioning programs or before the athlete begins strenuous activity. This allows the athlete to get back to play with a stronger and healthier body than before and again reduces the chance of injury.

- Computerized concussion baseline testing:
  - Purpose: Adequately assess the cognitive capabilities of the athlete
- Functional Neuro-Stabilization testing:
  - Purpose: Adequately assess the Neuro-Functional capabilities of the athlete such as:
    - Balance
    - Proprioception
    - Vestibulo-occular reflexes
- Functional Orthopedic testing
  - Purpose: Adequately assess the structural integrity of the muscles, bones and joints of the athlete, including:
  - Spine
  - Shoulders
  - Knees
  - Ankles

TREATMENT OF A CONCUSSION

Seek emergency care for anyone who experiences a head injury and:

- A loss of consciousness lasting more than a minute
- Repeated vomiting
- Seizures
- Obvious struggle with cognitive activity or physical coordination
- Symptoms that worsen over time

Once a patient has been evaluated by an Emergency Room or primary-care physician, they should then see a specialist in concussions to be further assessed so that the extent of the damage can be properly determined.

The Mayo Clinic says that it's inadvisable for athletes to return to play until the symptoms of the concussion are gone, *but indicates that a lack of symptoms does not mean that there is no injury, or that it does not require rehabilitation.* It just means that the most obvious signs of injury are no longer present. That is why I recommend patients seek the services of a professional for a more detailed analysis and neuro-rehabilitation.

Personally, I feel that resting is essential for patients who have had a concussion; real rest, not just bed for a day. This means no strenuous activities that may increase your heart rate or require physical lifting. Rest is a key factor because over-stimulation to an area of the brain that has been damaged can be harmful. Just like other injuries, the first step to treatment is rest.

You should also consider cutting down on other activities that can be *mentally* taxing, like working on the computer, watching TV, texting or playing video games.

When you are first checked by the doctor, he or she will do a neurological examination to evaluate the following:

- Memory and concentration
- Vision
- Hearing
- Strength and sensation
- Balance
- Coordination
- Reflexes

After that, if necessary, they may request a cranial computerized tomography (CT) which is a series of X-rays that will further evaluate the injury. This takes just a few minutes and is totally painless. The criteria used to determine whether or not the patient needs a CT scan are:

- You are an older adult.

- You fell from a height of more than 3 feet (1 meter).

- You were hit by a car or ejected from your car seat in a motor vehicle accident.

- You are under the influence of alcohol or drugs.

- You are unable to recall the incident for at least 30 minutes after it occurred.

- You have persistent difficulty with short-term memory—that is retaining new information—after you've completely regained consciousness.

- You have vomited several times.

- You had a seizure.

- You suffered bruises, scrapes or cuts on your head and neck.

- You are confused or have any other neurological symptoms, especially if those symptoms are getting worse.

If your injury is sufficiently severe, you might be kept in a hospital for observation. If not, the doctor will often send you home with instruction to have someone check on you every few hours. And that's about it! Unless something unfortunate happens as a result of the concussion, that's about all the doctors will do for you.

The treatment guidelines for concussions continue to evolve in terms of how long the physician should keep the athlete at rest and how many concussions within a season are acceptable. Because of these changing guidelines, I recommend physicians err on the side of caution, making sure that the brain is fully functioning before sending the young athlete back to play.

The concussion needs more than just a brief evaluation; the patient should be treated for the whole brain and not just for cognitive function. If other areas are damaged they must get the help, and, rest they need.

CONCUSSION CARE

Whatever your evaluation indicates, resting is always the first step. The next step is Neuro-functional rehabilitation. Just as you rehabilitate the body, you must rehabilitate the brain. After this type of injury, damage is repaired by stimulation, allowing for proper function over time. This is often the missing piece.

My personal suggestions regarding concussions are:

1. Treat a concussion like any other injury. If you sprain your ankle, let it rest to begin the healing process. For example, if you throw yourself right back into it, (which is tempting, I know) chronic ankle conditions may occur, especially if the ankle is not rehabbed properly. That could ruin your ankle permanently. If the ankle is not stimulated in the way it needs to be stimulated to start working again, then the first condition heals, but there are harmful effects moving forward because the ankle no longer works the same. The same is true for a concussion or any other traumatic brain injury, so take the time, *the first time*, to heal it properly, or risk that you may never function on the same level again. This holds true for any injury.

2. From there, it's essential to get rehabilitation measures started as soon as possible, to permit the best level of healing. Otherwise, it's like saying, "Okay; the ankle feels better, so let's put the patient back out on the field without rehabbing and see how it goes. What could go wrong?"

Would you like to gamble like that with your ankle? Probably not! Then, why would you do that with your brain and skull? That kind of reasoning doesn't make any sense and that's often the position that athletes are put in. Of course, we don't treat sprains that way.

On the other hand, the accepted approach, especially with concussions, is to rest the injury until you feel better and then go through a series of "back to play" protocol measures that are entirely symptom based. Then and only then can you get back into play.

While there are plenty of tools that help health care professionals to diagnose brain injury, there are few available treatment tools for this types of injuries. At this time, we have software that assists us in evaluating the return to play scenarios, but these are often limited in their capabilities and can be tricked. Nothing is guaranteed.

Often, athletes have "beaten" the computerized test by creating a cognitive baseline that is below what they can actually do. This allows them to go back to playing or performing, even after significant trauma; because the computer can't always assess the actual level of impairment.

While these programs are particularly helpful in returning an athlete to play, they are generally used as a major guide in the decision-making process. This "cheating" can be a pretty serious issue so personal and professional care should always be used in conjunction with this treatment tool.

A more in-depth approach is needed, but not often tried. Again, I must stress that it's just not enough to go to an ER or get a CAT scan, and then watch it over the next twelve hours and so on and so forth. You need the type of follow-up care that is rarely offered or even considered.

There are concussion specialists; that is, someone that has been specifically trained in functional neurology. These are the experts when it comes to this kind of brain injury. Practitioners trained by the Carrick Institute are excellent examples to look to and can determine whether the injury has diminished and if the brain is functioning to the point that the person can go back to normal activities. This is the same thought process that is used for any other injury such as the sprained ankle I mentioned. It's just a different procedure for assessment and treatment.

The fact is if you don't get proper treatment, and you're in a position for multiple concussions to happen, real damage can occur. The "gold standard" out there now is repeated evaluation, without any real care for the injured individuals. The lack of complete treatment options for concussions is really sad and I believe more development in thorough and proper treatment is absolutely necessary to prevent further or permanent brain injury in these cases.

STEPS to Concussion Care:

- Rest
- Functional Neurological Assessment
- Neurological Rehabilitation
    - Vestibulo-Occular Exercises
    - Balance and Coordination Exercises
    - Cognitive Training
- Re-evaluation of Functional Neurological Assessment
- Possible additional Neuro Rehab
- Return to play Sequence
- Return to Play

A CASE STUDY IN CONCUSSIONS:

A 16 year old teen-aged baseball player presented 3 weeks post-concussion. He was grazed by a ball being hit back up the middle; he was a team pitcher. He had already been released back to play by his family physician and had passed his impact test.

The weird thing is, his he presented with blurry vision when trying to hold gaze on the catcher's mitt and he had not been hit since the accident. Therefore, he should not have been released back to pitching. He was concerned because they had a regional tournament the following weekend.

After a comprehensive examination, he was found to have nystagmus while trying to track with his eyes, horizontally to the right. He was also unable to fixate his gaze when his eyes were in a downward position. He had an altered gait pattern and balance issue while standing with his eyes closed and both feet together.

Implementing very specific chiropractic manipulative therapy, along with eye movement exercises and basic stabilization work, dedicated to one side of the body only, the young pitcher was then released with at-home exercises that he was to perform 5 times per day for 15 seconds each time.

Upon the follow-up visit two days later, the blurry vision was gone and the balance was back to normal. He was re-evaluated and it was determined that he continued to have slight nystagmus with eyes tracking. He was given one additional exercise to be performed 5 times per day for 10 seconds and was to return for follow-up in 4 days.

Upon his return, all signs and symptoms were no longer present. He was returned to play at the appropriate time. He played the regional tournament that weekend and went 5-6 at the plate and did not let up a run in the 4 innings he pitched.

Chapter 6

Nutrition for Sports

Too often poor nutrition indirectly causes injury and this type of injury is not the type to just go away all by itself, after the fact. These are the injuries that linger and may never allow you to feel the same again.

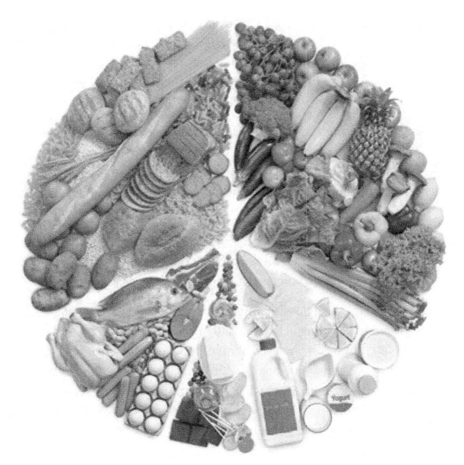

PROPER NUTRITION & PREVENTION

Let's get started with the most basic step in nutrition: **Food.**

We all must eat -- right? And, if you're an athlete, you probably know that what you eat is fundamentally important. But just how important is it?

Making sure you eat the right foods could be more crucial than you know. If you don't have the right nutrients in your body to recover after exercise or injury, then the tissue won't repair properly and that may lead to a myriad of problems. If the tissue doesn't heal properly, then it can't perform at its optimum, and you can't perform at your optimum ... and that's essentially what you want.

Then, when it's time for you to try to push through your routine exercises, you could end up hurting yourself. Damaged tissue means that you have an injury that means, when it comes to food, getting what you need and getting it at the right time, and in the right form, can help you avoid this problem from becoming long-term and chronic.

Generally, the impact of good food on your health is often a neglected subject when, in fact, it should be a corner stone of your routine. As an athlete, your body demands certain nutrients so that you can perform at your best. That being said, don't go out and grab the first diet plan you see.

Everyone is uniquely different —athletes included. What works for one person, one sport, or one training program may not work for another. I think that having a customized nutritional program is your best bet, assuring that the program is tailored to your specific nutritional needs.

Often, athletes struggle with food requirements and figuring out exactly what they should be eating before and after exercise or sports performances. Those who are physically involved should know exactly what kind of food to prime their systems with before, during and after strenuous exertion. Specifically, they need to know what foods are required for recovery and cellular repair. Often poor nutrition is the indirect cause of injury, leading to incomplete healing and even chronic inflammation.

Whether, you're a baseball pitcher with a bad shoulder, a runner with a trick knee, or a football player with a concussion … **chronic inflammation is your enemy.**

KNOW WHAT YOU ARE EATING

Understanding what you are eating is something that many people seem to struggle with due to the vast amount of nutritional misinformation (otherwise known as dietary propaganda) that's put out there before the public. Most of the facts and statistics that are on the glossy brochures, or the well-designed product packaging include paid testimonials specifically written for mass-marketing. Well-placed advertisements that we find online and in print increase our belief that what they are saying is as good as gospel.

One example of this is the explosion of popularity in Greek yogurt, supposedly because it has more protein than other yogurt. But, have you ever evaluated the sugar content of yogurt? It's actually about the same as a candy bar.

Another example of this is the glut of protein bars on the market. Look at the high sugar and carbohydrate content, as well as the low quality of protein within the bars. Again, it's not much better than eating a candy bar.

THINK DIFFERENTLY ABOUT NUTRITION

From my life experience, my education and my Chiropractic healthcare practice, I have a very different concept about nutrition and weight control. I'm not a calorie counter at all, because:

- You are not a serving size.
- You are not the number that pops up on a scale.

Those things are really immaterial in determining the proper calculation of food for you to consume in order to have excellent health.

My nutritional philosophy is simply quality over quantity. I really do believe, and I see it every day, that you can put large quantities of the right nutrients into your body. If your body can efficiently absorb, utilize, metabolize and expel the waste product, your weight will not increase.

The problem with calories begins when you put the wrong calories into your body. The proverbial "empty calorie" is what I am speaking about.

WHAT'S AN EMPTY CALORIE

An empty calorie is one that lacks nutritional value. No nutritional value means that you don't get any of the necessary macronutrients or micronutrients out the food you just ate.

If you have never read Michael Pollen's books, please pick them up; they are eye openers for most of us.

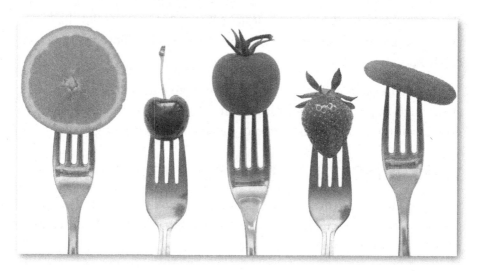

Food

noun, often attributive \'füd\

a: *material consisting essentially of protein, carbohydrate, and fat used in the body of an organism to sustain growth, repair, and vital processes and to furnish energy; also: such food together with supplementary substances (as minerals, vitamins, and condiments).*
Credit: http://www.merriam-webster.com/ dictionary/ food?show=0&t=1372164149

In the most basic sense, food for human consumption is comprised of macronutrients, (carbohydrates, fats, and proteins) and micronutrients, (vitamins and minerals) and water. And, that's all!

Micronutrients are usually lacking in the best tasting food we eat, as well as the junk food we consume.

Carbohydrates (carbs for short) are foods that provide us with energy by being converted to sugar (glucose) in our bodies. That's all they do for us.

In the 1980s, there was this enormous low fat + high carbohydrate push in the United States. "Fats were making us fat and causing heart disease" is what everyone was saying. Err, we were wrong!

Fats don't make you fat, although they can in excess, but if they are the wrong fats, they most certainly will. Carbs make you fat if you eat way too many and then can't burn off enough of them through physical activity. What doesn't get used up gets converted to sugar, which is then stored as fat.

LET ME ASK A QUESTION, AND THEN ANSWER IT.

How many carbs do you need for a single day?
Technically, none!

Now, don't go crazy and cut them out of your diet all together, especially if you are an athlete. What I said before is true; our bodies can get along just fine without carbohydrates. The only problem is our brain l-o-v-e-s those sugars one heck of a lot.

Your brain, which is the central processing unit of the body, is the Captain of your ship, but it's a sugar junkie. In fact, 30-40% of the glucose used by your body is used by your three-pound brain. If you weigh 200 lbs., then 1.5% of your body weight (although it is the most important 1.5%) uses 30-40% of that sugar produced.

FATS

Fats are critical to your health and well-being, and obviously should be the highest quality fats such as Omega 3, 6, 7, and 9 which are extremely healthy and necessary for human health. Saturated and Trans-fatty acids are extremely unhealthy and unnecessary for our bodies. Both are fats, but there is a distinct difference.

Good fats are fundamentally essential fatty acids. To keep it simple, Omega 3, 6, 7, and 9 and unsaturated fats are beneficial for our bodies.

HOW CAN FAT CAN BE BENEFICIAL FOR US

The membranes of our cells are a double layer of fat, (phospholipid bilayer). The good kind of fats helps us repair and generate new cell membranes, keeping cells healthy and/or regenerating new healthy cells. Omega 3 fatty acids are actually anti-inflammatory. Inflammation (there's that word again) is the subject of common concern in nutrition. Omega 3 fats can also be used by our bodies as a nutrient rich energy source.

Bad fats that are in our system are harmful, just as good fats are beneficial. If your body uses the wrong types of fats for cell membrane repair or regeneration, then the new or regenerated cell membrane will be fragile. Weak cell membranes lead to the early demise of the cell. Early demise of the cell leads to increased demand for cell regeneration or cell turnover. Cell turnover is also known as the aging process.

Is aging bad? Well, not really. However, premature aging of your body certainly is not a pleasant thing. So, the right kinds of fats are healthy and excellent for your body. They allow you to have healthy repair and regeneration of cells, decrease bodily inflammation and they provide you with high quality, long term energy.

The wrong kinds of fats can be horrible to our bodies. They lead to premature cell death, aging, inflammation and are generally not healthy for us in any way.

PROTEIN

Ah, the all mighty protein! Nothing is better than protein when we're talking sports nutrition, right?

Well, the answer is actually yes and no. *Yes,* in the sense of repairing your muscle tissue that breaks down during exercise, increasing your immune system's ability to repair and fight infection and helping you provide energy when your bodies need it.

No, in the sense that most athletes take in way too much protein. Too much protein is hard on your kidneys and quite frankly, too much is not used efficiently or effectively in any way.

The building blocks of proteins are amino acids. Let's call amino acids the nutrient components of proteins. Amino acids can be absorbed and utilized by our bodies in a number of ways. There are 22 known amino acids, 9 of which are "essential". Essential amino acids are ones that ***must*** be ingested.

Our bodies can actually create the other 13 by utilizing different pathways of the body. You'd be very surprised how many ways different amino acids are used by your body. These uses include hormone precursors, brain chemicals, tissue repair, immune support, liver enzymatic activity, energy production, etc… the list goes on and on.

Essential	Nonessential
Histidine	Alanine
Isoleucine	Arginine
Leucine	Asparagine
Lysine	Aspartic acid
Methionine	Cysteine
Phenylalanine	Glutamic acid
Threonine	Glutamine
Tryptophan	Glycine
Valine	Ornithine
	Proline
	Serine
	Tyrosine

MICRONUTRIENTS

Some people take multivitamins believing that doing so will help them nutritionally, and to some degree it does. However, the amount of the vitamins that actually gets absorbed into the system varies significantly from product to product.

The typical one-a-day multivitamin is virtually useless. Some healthcare professionals would suggest that you are just manufacturing extremely expensive urine and, although I feel that this idea is generally ignorant, it's true when you are dealing with most off-the-shelf multivitamin products. You don't typically feel better after taking your multivitamin, however, the micronutrient content that you should be getting from a multi-vitamin is just as vital to you as the macronutrient content of your body. Finding quality multi-vitamins that your body can absorb properly is the key.

Micronutrients are nutrients that our body uses, but only in small amounts. These include vitamins, minerals, and other trace compounds that are necessary to sustain life. In fact, they are more important than most people realize because they are the catalysts for certain chemical processes to exist in our bodies.

In chemistry, or biochemistry, a catalyst is a substance that allows, drives or changes the speed of a chemical reaction. Without catalysts to support those biochemical reactions in our bodies, we wouldn't exist. Most of us have seen someone, at least once in our lives, who was malnourished, and the first impression we have is that they need to eat, which is obvious.

But, the real danger is that they are probably missing some essential micronutrients that their body requires, and that can cause them to become seriously ill or die.

This relates to how people eat. My job, in all of this, is to help patients and athletes change their food habits. One example of this is moving from eating one meal a day to eating multiple meals over the course of a day. Eating healthful nutritious food is the key, instead of food that does not contain the nutrients that a healthy body needs and craves.

SPACED MEALS THROUGHOUT THE DAY

I am a firm believer that you will be better off by consistently eating throughout the day, every two to three hours, and consuming quality foods that keep your body metabolizing and utilizing nutrients. Thus, you are constantly fueling your system to repair and become healthier and never overfilling your tank at one sitting.

I also help my patients hold themselves accountable for getting the correct education about what is excellent and not so good in the area of nutrition for their bodies.

As I mentioned early on, there's a lot of misinformation out there; tons of websites, blogs, and books. Everyone has different perspectives and opinions. My perspective is that there is no one best way. *Do what works for you for optimal health and optimum performance,* because what works for you won't necessarily work for everyone, even though the basic concepts may be the same.

I believe there is another element that makes my approach as a chiropractor unique; being open to the right path and holding patients accountable for their own health and well-being through nutrition. A large part of sports coaching and the athlete's performance equates to a special lifestyle and healthy mindset. There are tremendous advantages when you figure out exactly what your body needs through empirical testing.

FOOD MANAGEMENT THROUGH A NUTRITIONAL PROGRAM

The next important thing is using the proper nutritional program. That means employing the right approach for you and staying on task, whether it's food, exercise, management skills or whatever is necessary for you, the patient or athlete to achieve the desired results.

What's tricky is, it's not something that you can simply find in a book. It's something that is most effectively developed by an expert and it can, over the long term, work for you without having to be coached. It's a lifestyle that you need to design and develop with a professional. There is a way to create it. Most people don't have the capacity to initiate that process on their own, and that's some thing else that I'm here to help you with.

THE THREE MAIN COMPONENTS TO SPORTS NUTRITION

1. The ability to produce energy.
2. The potential to reduce the amount of damage that your body endures.
3. The ability to provide your body with the potential to heal properly.

When we engage in sports or any physically strenuous activity, we break down and rebuild muscle tissue. We metabolize nutrients, and we expel waste products. These three factors are vital to our body's performance.

ENERGY PRODUCTION

Producing energy mainly depends on eating the right foods at the right times. There are a lot of energy drinks and energy supplements on the market today. In my opinion, it is best to stay away from these drinks and supplements because, essentially, they are stimulants.

Stimulants are certainly not energy producers, and there is a vast difference between the two. Energy nutrients allow your body to produce energy; stimulants do not!

Using stimulants forces your body to quickly produce hormones that accelerate your nervous system and can lead to a multitude of harmful short and long-term side effects. Some stimulants can cause increased heart rate, anxiety and insomnia. They are dangerous to your physical and mental well being; they deregulate your hormonal balance and in the long run they will damage your ability to produce energy on your own.

These products are never for continued use as most of them contain caffeine. Caffeine is a central nervous system stimulant and studies show that caffeine often mitigates the effects of sleep deprivation and increases performance during a very short period of interval training. If you are going to use caffeine-based stimulates, use them wisely, and never on a daily basis.

Another element to energy production is your ability to train properly to make sure that you're not overstraining yourself. This is essential to ensure your body is not breaking down tissue too aggressively. Listen to your body, train with a plan and make a commitment not to over-train, which could reduce energy production and increase tissue breakdown.

EAT THE RIGHT FOODS

The basic instruction I give is to eat high quality foods and high quality nutrients. In terms of energy production, high-quality foods would be foods with the proper nutrients that help your body produce energy-packing fuel for your body's optimum performance.

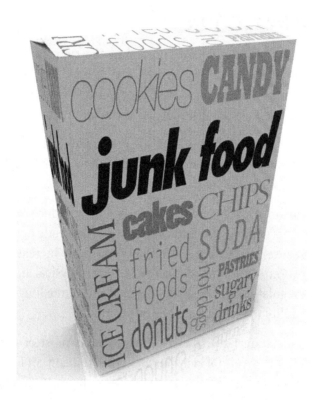

JUNK FOOD ISN'T FOOD - IT'S GARBAGE

Junk food isn't even food; it's correctly called junk food for a good reason. Junk food is anything that is highly processed, either plastic packaged or comes in a box, and is actually engineered to sit on a shelf almost indefinitely. It may have artificial flavor, color, and color or flavor enhancers as well as a lot of preservatives.

It might be fast food, from a big chain, fast-food restaurant or any type of food product that has added sugar, added salt.

Just because you chew and consume something doesn't mean it is food. Junk food cannot effectively generate energy for our bodies. It really comes down to eating only high-quality foods and eating at the right times if you want to successfully generate energy for your body. There are also supplements and programs that you can use to increase energy production.

RAW FOOD DIETS

In terms of the right kinds of foods, some foods can be raw foods but not necessarily all of them should be raw. Your foods simply must be foods that have high-quality nutrient components that your body can break down, use and then excrete the waste from, properly.

Healthy foods, like fruits and vegetables specifically, green leafy vegetables, and lean, high-quality protein like fish, turkey, some grain-fed organic beef, even some organic pork, are all examples of high quality foods. Steer clear of processed foods and refined sugars – period!

HOW ENERGY IS PRODUCED BY THE CELLS

Your mitochondria are the energy producers of your cellular structure. The energy currency for the work that animals must do is the energy-rich molecule known as adenosine triphosphate (ATP). The ATP is produced by the mitochondria using the energy that you have stored from your food intake.

A typical animal cell will have about 1,000 to 2,000 mitochondria. So the cell will have a lot of structures capable of producing a large quantity of available energy. This ATP production by the mitochondria is done through your respiration process, which is essentially the use of oxygen to generate energy. This is a very effective method for using food energy to make ATP.

One of the benefits of "aerobic exercise" is that it improves your body's ability to make ATP quickly using breathing. In order for the mitochondria to produce ATP, there is a process called the Citric Acid Cycle. This is a fairly long and complicated process, but what is essential is the need for Ubiquinone as a key component for this process to occur. (Ubiquinone is also known as Co-Enzyme-Q10). This compound is typically produced by the body unless you are taking statin drugs, (cholesterol medication). Statin drugs block an enzyme called HMG CO-A Reductase. This enzyme is necessary for cholesterol production in your body and is also needed for production of Ubiquinone by the body. A serious side effect of statin drugs is physical fatigue.

All living cells have mitochondria. Some cells have more mitochondria than others. However, the cells of our hair and outer skin cells are already dead and no longer produce ATP.

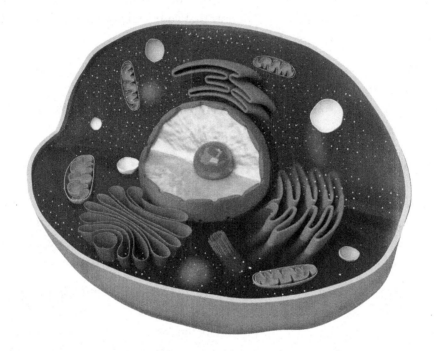

YOUR EATING SCHEDULE

The best time of the day for you to eat, should be based upon eating unusually small frequent meals, containing only high-quality foods. In terms of sports performance, priming comes anywhere between four hours to a half-hour before an event, training or practice. Be sure you're taking in higher carbohydrate-rich meals all the way up to 30 to 60 minutes before your athletic performance.

During training and exercise, your-body requires an intake of carbs and protein at about a 4 to 1 ratio by weight consumption. During recovery after exercise, training, or an event, a carbohydrate to protein ratio of about 2 to 1 is more appropriate.

EATING FOR RECOVERY

Optimal recovery requires that you are eating the right recovery foods within that 45 to 60-minute window of opportunity. Make sure the carbohydrates to protein ratio is correct – 2:1. Some research indicates that you have about two hours of time to take in the right nutrients for recovery, but my recommendation is that it would be best for you to keep it to under 1-hour, post exercise.

It is recommended that you develop the desire for and a lifestyle that includes mostly complex carbohydrates, high quality fats and lean high-quality proteins. You can easily achieve this by getting added supplements through a protein shake or a high-quality medical food.

Included in optimal recovery is rest in-between training sessions. Then high-quality sleep (a deep, sound sleep on a bed with a good firm mattress for 7-9 hours every night). During your sleep cycle, your body gets the opportunity to heal and repair without disruption from activities.

The result is the next day you can perform at your best once again.

NUTRITIONAL TIMING

When	Timing
Priming	Eat a high carbohydrate meal 4 hours before event or exercise. This often results in improved performance. Consume carbohydrates 60 min. before exercise as this also improves performance.
During	Exercise and events lasting longer than an hour: Consume 10-15 grams of carbohydrates every 15 min. Liquid consumption is typically best. A mixture of types of sugars appears to be beneficial. Carbs:Protein should be 4:1.
Recovery	Consumption should take place 45-60 min max. Combine carbs and protein at ratio of 2:1. Example: 200 lb. athlete: 30-40 grams/carbs and 15-20 grams/proteins.

Nutrition timing varies between athletes and between sports. One key underlying factor is your fluid intake. Water is your primary liquid in sports and in life. I recommend 64 oz. for children and 96 oz. for adults per day. Sports drinks are added to the 64-96 oz. requirement. Consumption of water during exercise or event is also essential.

FLUIDS

I want to make this topic as simple and easy as possible to learn. Your body is like a plant; it's producing cells every day, and it must have water every day. Drink water and avoid dehydration at all costs. It's unsuitable for performance when you dehydrate, but more importantly it's devastating for your health.

DEHYDRATION

Dehydration is the loss of fluids from the body. It can either be loss of blood volume or fluid volume from within the cells itself. Water is crucial to almost all bodily functions, and the loss of even 2% of our body's water is high risk.

As a population, we are already chronically dehydrated. It is possible to drink too much water without proper electrolytes, but the state of dehydration that most of us are in, mixed with the amount of sodium we eat, makes this unlikely. However, don't drink excessive amounts of water quickly because it can lead to other issues, as well.

The three main modes of excretion of waste from your body include:

- Urination
- Defecation
- Perspiration

All of these functions are highly dependent on the hydration of your body. Be sure to drink 96 oz. of water every day.

If you are dehydrated, eliminating the waste products from your bodily "plant" (the power plant inside of you that creates energy) becomes quite limited and varies in performance from remarkably slow – to extremely fast and highly dangerous.

A major factor to consider is that your optimum performance and toxicity do not mix. The better condition your elimination system is in the greater your capacity for the elimination of bodily wastes in a safe way. This also provides a greater capacity for properly utilizing nutrients in the body.

Just as you take in oxygen and eliminate carbon dioxide through breathing, so your body takes in nutrients and produces waste products that must be eliminated. Water is the main ingredient in making this happen efficiently. Water is the essential system lubricant.

ELECTROLYTES

Let's just say, for the purpose of this book, that electrolytes may be defined as compounds that break apart (ionize) when dissolved in water. The main ions that are physiologically used by your body are:

- Sodium (Na)
- Potassium (K)
- Calcium (Ca)
- Magnesium (Mg)
- Chlorine (Cl)

Basically, what electrolytes do in our bodies is govern the distribution of fluid in and on the exterior of our cells. Nutrients and other compounds circulate in the body's water, into and out of the cell structure. If there is an imbalance, those cells will not receive the proper nutrient levels. They would, then, have a more difficult time ridding the body of waste from within each cell.

This fluid balance is critical for your body's ability to control the pH level of your blood. The pH of the blood is very tightly regulated and essential to cell survival. Even small fluctuations of pH in the blood can be dangerous and result in cell demise.

HYDRATION & SPORTS PERFORMANCE

Aerobic athletes such as marathon runners, gymnasts, tri-athletes and strength/power athletes such as sprinters or football players, all have different hydration requirements during performance.

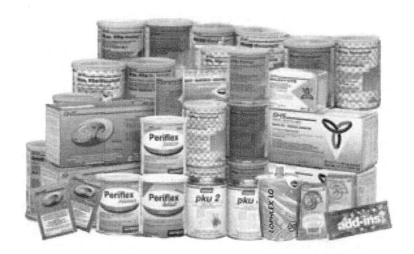

MEDICAL FOODS

What I call "medical" foods are actually foods that function as meal replacements and are intended to relieve an underlying health-related condition. They contain vital nutrients that are specific to the problem that has been identified as the issue, and that is almost always inflammation.

There are a few select, high-quality supplement companies who offer more medically-oriented, pharmaceutical grade supplements and higher-quality products that are geared towards correcting clinical symptoms.

In my own training regimen, I take a medical food incorporated into my post work out shake to reduce any inflammation in my system. I also take a very high-quality supplement and medical food to support my liver and digestive tract. I add fiber to that shake and dark greens or an exceptionally concentrated deep green product.

THE SUPPLEMENT MARKET IS NOT REGULATED

The FDA has no control over supplements. What this means is that what is on the label of the supplement can be either misleading or frankly, false. When trying to find the right medical food and supplement, always be sure it has a GMP certification (Good Manufacturing Practices). This certification is one way for the industry to regulate itself. This certification is extremely expensive to get and extremely difficult to maintain, but the consumer knows that the company is putting their money into their products and making sure that their product labeling is truthful and accurate.

One of the best ways to get exceptionally high-quality products is to talk with a natural healthcare doctor who has access to the products and can order them for you.

The other advantage of going through your healthcare professional is that they know exactly what you need, specific for your body. Sprinters should be eating and training differently than marathon runners; these athletes should be eating and training differently than strength trainers, who should be eating and training differently than volleyball players. Everyone has unique needs for their body and their sport, so you may want to work with someone specifically trained to help with your professional sport needs.

I would consider these people Health Coaches, (I will go more in-depth about health coaching in a later chapter). These types of coaches/health professionals work with some of the best athletes in the world and virtually all athletes have sports coaches:

Tiger Woods has a swing coach, and he's one of the best golfers in the world.

Michael Jordan had a basketball coach, and he was the best basketball player in the world.

So, even the highest performing people still need coaches or individuals that can manage, improve and refine their ability to perform at their best. That's where health coaching can play a significant role regarding health improvement for optimum performance.

REDUCING DAMAGE & PREVENTING FREE RADICALS

Cellular damage occurs because of free-radical activity and inflammation. This is when the body breaks down, often when you're exercising, and you break down tissue. When this occurs, you're really metabolizing high-quality nutrients into waste product. If you're not processing waste products properly, they damage the cells and the body. When that damage occurs, the body then has to repair those cells and energy is needlessly redirected toward the process of repairing cells.

You can decrease cellular damage by taking supplements and eating foods containing high-quality antioxidants like Selenium, Coenzyme Q10, Vitamin C, and Vitamin E. Basically, fruits and vegetables with deep and bright colors are especially loaded with antioxidants. Antioxidants donate electrons to the cells, which neutralize free-radicals that are damaging to cellular tissue.

DETOXIFICATION

Buzz word; DETOX! You cannot buy a detox off the shelf. OK, they do sell things called detox, but let me warn you about them. Don't buy them! You've been warned.

There is a misconception that has been created by marketing professionals. Detoxification takes place in your body through the liver, so supporting this process is important. However, most of the detoxification products being sold are just junk. It is best to work with a healthcare professional to detoxify your body safely and effectively. Detoxification is unquestionably not a one-size-fits-all approach.

You must first know if the gastrointestinal tract is working properly before undertaking detoxification. You need to know that your intestinal tract is absorbing and utilizing nutrients correctly, that the lymph system is draining properly, that the liver is working as it should and that the kidneys are filtering appropriately. A detox off the shelf will not take care of your needs - I've warned you again!

INTESTINAL PERMEABILITY ISSUES "Leaky Gut"

Intestinal Permeability is a significant source of toxic load and a significant cause of inflammation. Chronic inflammation causes disease in our bodies, and plays the central role in many diseases that we believe to be age related, i.e. heart disease, high cholesterol, arthritis, autoimmune disorders, and neurologic disorders.

The small intestine is the digestive/absorptive organ for nutrients, as well as a powerful, mechanical immunity barrier against excessive absorption of bacteria, food antigens, and other macromolecules.

Both mal-absorption and increased intestinal permeability ("leaky gut") are associated with chronic gastrointestinal imbalances as well as many systemic disorders.

Intestinal Permeability refers to the permeability of the small intestine; the higher the permeability, the more problems it can cause in the body. The issue is that increased permeability also increases the number of foreign compounds entering the bloodstream, which is then shuttled directly to the liver. The vast majority of the blood supply to the liver comes from the digestive tract, through the hepatic portal vein. This transports anything that crosses the digestive barrier to the liver, to be differentiated and dealt with appropriately. If the liver is unable to deal with the substances appropriately, the first stage of liver detoxification is to tag molecules to make them fat-soluble. This allows for storage of the waste product in fat cells as opposed to elimination.

YO-YO DIETING AND LEAKY GUT

It is very difficult to reduce body fat when having intestinal permeability issues. This is one of the major causes of yo-yo dieting and why most people have remarkably little chance of being successful with weight loss in the long run. This also goes back to the concept that quality of nutrients is far more important than quantity of calories.

People suffering from leaky gut syndrome have a higher risk of their small intestine allowing entry of bacterial antigens (capable of cross-reacting with host tissue to enter the bloodstream), leading to autoimmune process problems. This also allows for the uptake of toxic compounds that can overwhelm the hepatic (liver) detoxification process, and leads to an overly sensitive immune system.

Here are some symptoms of Leaky Gut Syndrome, but make no mistake; an increase in inflammation in the body degrades the weakest link in your health. The following list is just a synopsis of the issues that these patients experience:

- Heart Disease
- Arthritis
- Fibromyalgia
- Fatigue (Chronic and Otherwise)
- Obesity
- Low Libido
- Hormonal Issues
- Diabetes
- Inflammatory Bowel Disease (IBD)
- Food allergies
- Inflammatory joint disease
- Chronic dermatologic conditions

Research shows that the increased permeability observed in patients with ankylosing spondylitis, rheumatoid arthritis, and vasculitis may be an influential factor in the detrimental effects of these disorders.

On the other side of the equation, decreased permeability is an underlying principle of mal-absorption, subsequent malnutrition and failure to thrive. In certain disease states of the small intestine, such as gluten-sensitive enteropathy, permeability to large molecules may increase while permeability to small molecules decreases; a result of damage to the microvilli.

This is associated with Celiac Disease. As a result, nutrients become even less accessible to assist in the detoxification of antigens flooding the system.

There are a number of possible causes of intestinal permeability, such as:

- Antibiotic usage
- Intestinal infection
- Ingestion of allergenic foods or toxic chemicals
- Deficient secretory IgA
- Trauma and endotoxemia
- NSAIDs, anti-inflammatory drugs such as Ibuprofen, Naproxen

NON-INVASIVE EXAM FOR LEAKY GUT SYNDROME

The good news is that an examination for Leaky Gut Syndrome called Intestinal Permeability Assessment is a noninvasive assessment of small intestinal absorption and barrier function in the bowel. The procedure measures the ability of two non-metabolized sugar molecules to penetrate the intestinal mucosa.

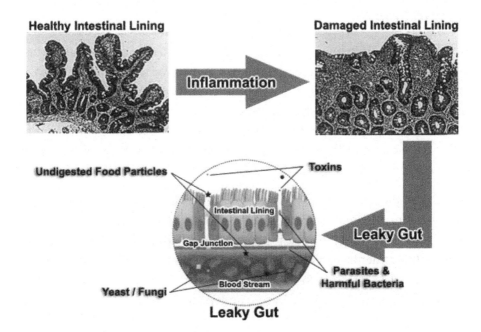

Leaky Gut

Before a person takes the test, they are asked to stop certain medications that could interfere with the results of the exam. Also, they must not eat or drink anything 8 hours before the evaluation. Often, their healthcare professional will also make sure that their fasting glucose level is not too high.

WEIGHT LOSS AND TOXINS

Weight loss can be difficult because there are so many waste products and toxins in body fat, which the body must handle when they come out. If the body can't handle it, the athlete's/patient's performance suffers significantly. They're fatigued. They're toxic. They have brain fog.

This is another reason to work with a health coach, to monitor a detox program. A weight loss program is a detoxification program of sorts, which can be critically damaging to your health if done incorrectly. How many people touting weight loss programs actually understand the body, detoxification, intestinal permeability, inflammation, and chronic illness? Remarkably, the answer is very few. Utilize a trusted healthcare professional; it will save you a lot of hassle, unnecessary suffering and, for that matter, money.

TOXIC LOAD

I believe that junk food and processed foods are environmental toxins. Toxins are poisons that the body must convert to waste and excrete. Toxins are shown to reduce the body's ability to produce energy at a cellular level. Junk foods are toxins within our system, and our bodies try to use and convert them into usable nutrients for cellular repair, energy production and other processes. The body struggles with processing things like artificial sweeteners and trans-fatty acids.

Our bodies must try to process these toxins through the liver and then excrete them. The more your body is wasting energy trying to perform this activity, the less energy it has for the actual completion of any sports activity, work activity, mental challenges, stress challenges or cellular repair. Each of these becomes a load that the body just does not have the energy required to handle because the body is operating under a toxic load.

Your body is like a car. If you put faulty gas in it, its performance is going to decrease drastically. It's like putting sugar in the gas tank. Sugar will destroy a car and it destroys the body in much the same fashion. In summary, it is quality of nutrition over quantity of nutrition — hands down.

NUTRIENT DEMANDS ON THE BODY IF IT GETS INJURED

The nutrient demand on a simple musculoskeletal injury increases by at least 20 to 25 percent. An injured person will need to increase their proteins as they synthesize proteins to make immunoglobulins. With the correct type and quantity of nutrients, your immune system can actually work properly to break down the damaged tissue and/or repair tissue to a normal, healthy state.

Improper healing and remodeling of tissue would be considered scar tissue. Scar tissue does not have the same physical properties as normal tissue and, therefore, does not let the body perform in the same manner.

Trauma, whether it's skeletal or otherwise, such as a sprained ankle, an injured back, a broken arm, or whatever it may be, imposes one of the highest load demands on energy utilization. So, without a doubt, you must increase energy production in all ways possible when you are injured.

During times of injury or trauma, our energy demands go up, and our need for cellular synthesis goes up as well. We must remove damaged tissue through waste elimination and replace it with new, healthy tissue.

THE TWO TO FOUR WEEK WINDOW

There is a two to four week window, known as the acute/sub-acute phases. The acute phase (1st and 2nd week) is critical for removal of some injured tissue and for beginning of repair work for damaged tissue. During the sub-acute phase (3rd and 4th week), the body is repairing and remodeling new tissue that is to be used by the body for healing. If the injury is muscular in nature, the body remodels muscle tissue in this phase.

These first four weeks are clearly the most critical to the long-term injury outcome. This is why you should seek treatment immediately if you are injured. If you start to remodel muscle using scar tissue, your performance will decrease.

We've mentioned this earlier; scar tissue doesn't have the same contractile force as muscle tissue. It doesn't have the same stretch-ability or pliability, and you are liable to experience another injury while your performance continues to decline. This is why it is so important to address nutritional demands directly after injury. This acute/sub-acute phase is a critical time when the immune system clearly needs to be supported. The injury also needs to be treated properly and promptly to reduce the risk of the acute injury becoming chronic.

What happens in the acute and sub-acute phases is that the body requires more minerals and vitamins to accommodate the demands of handling the injury. It uses those nutrients to activate the immune system, increase the rate of protein synthesis and increase the rate of cellular proliferation or synthesis. In the exceptionally acute phase when the tissue is broken down, energy levels must increase to handle healing.

According to Dr. Bob Rakowski, the protein synthesis requirements of trauma --based on the skeletal system – are almost the same as what they would be for a burn. Therefore, your body actually goes into a highly specific response that requires a lot of energy (a lot of protein synthesis) and requires your immune system to be supported when there's trauma involved.

During the four to eight week window, the body is laying down the new tissue and creating a neurologic and nutritional support for the new tissue. So not only is the healthy tissue created, but the way the brain utilizes and coordinates the utilization of that tissue is determined.

The six to eight week window is particularly crucial to regain proper use of damaged tissue for different reasons all together. This phase of care needs to focus on rehabilitation and retraining the body and brain to utilize that new tissue, and typically requires less energy expenditure.

PROPER SUPPLEMENTS ARE ESSENTIAL FOR HEALING – A REVIEW

Few companies genuinely manufacture high-quality supplements, and those are typically sold to physicians. Therefore, your physician's office is the best place to get the quality supplements. You and those supplements should be GMP certified. Supplements, in general, are essential in this day and age, not only to help athletes perform at an extremely high level, but to support average healthy individuals as well.

Our food supply and the way we grow, produce and package our food severely limits the quantity of actual, high-quality nutritional value that can be obtained by eating it. Even when we select lean meats, we are still likely dealing with the potential use of antibiotics and steroids to produce the fatter cow, thus increasing profitability for the ranchers.

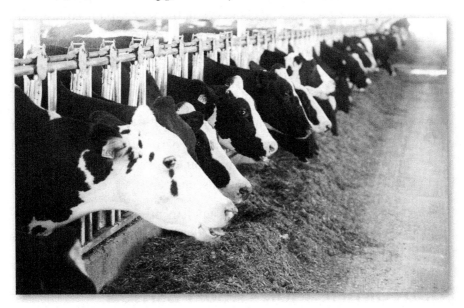

When we purchase fruits and vegetables, unless they are certified organic, we are probably introducing toxic chemicals into our body, including pesticides and herbicides.

High-quality fats include fish oil, and the toxic load is determined by whatever contaminants the fish were swimming in. Traditionally, this is considered eating "lean and clean": eating fruit, vegetables, lean proteins and high-quality fats.

The method by which our food supply is currently produced limits our ability to get the nutrients out of our food, again, not just for performance but to live healthy lives.

If you're an athlete, you have a much higher demand for energy production and tissue repair. Supplements, then, become even more critical to get all the fats, carbohydrates, proteins, vitamins, minerals and water that you need for your higher energy demand.

INCORRECT ASSUMPTIONS

It's a mistake to assume that you could get all the water you need just from eating food, without drinking any water at all. It's the same mistake to believe that you're going to get all the vitamins, minerals and macronutrients that you need by eating food without taking supplements. Although it is possible, it is very unlikely that this will occur.

Nutritional absorption is highly influenced by the state of health of your gastrointestinal tract. If you have issues such as permeability issues, leaky gut issues, underlying infections or inflammation, these conditions are going to limit your ability to absorb and utilize those nutrients properly.

Furthermore, if you use low-quality supplements, be aware that they are typically filled with binders and other ingredients that don't enable the body to break them down for proper nutritional use. Be forewarned!

FOOD FORTIFICATION – A SUPPOSITION

Suppose I am a dairy producer and I have to add fortifications of Calcium to my milk; the first question any wise milk drinker should ask is, "Why would you have to fortify milk with Calcium. Doesn't milk already contain Calcium?" As the producer, I'm not required to put on the carton packaging what chemical compound of Calcium is being used to bolster the milk.

The next question should be "What chemical form of Calcium do you use to fortify the milk?"

From a financial perspective, the dairy producer is going to use the cheapest form of Calcium that he can legally get away with using.

Last question, "Is the chemical make-up of the Calcium used the most efficient and effective for the absorption and utilization of Calcium in my body?"

And, of course that last question is the big one; usually-the chemical is not that efficiently absorbed and utilized by the body.

Now, this scenario may not be 100% accurate, but it's worth thinking about, and it gives us an easy example of what fortified means when you see it on food packaging.

WHAT <u>ENRICHED</u> AND <u>FORTIFIED</u> REALLY MEAN

The terms enriched and fortified in the food world are a gold mine to the industry and a curse for the consumer.

You believe that you're eating something nutritious and actually you are unwittingly increasing the toxic load on your body.

What the food industry is doing is removing the high-quality nutrients, adding poor, lower-quality, cheaper nutrients, and your body doesn't utilize them properly.

The same is true for supplements. Since they are not regulated, the quality standard for supplements isn't about quality at all. What the supplement company claims is in the bottle may not be in there at all, or the formulation of the compound may be cheap and non-absorbable. Unfortunately, it's more about their bottom line than your health.

For example, there are different compounds that are all considered Vitamin C, but they are not all equally absorbed and utilized by the body.

This is another reason working with a professional, with access to known reputable "nutraceutical" companies, is essential. That doesn't mean that you can only get high quality supplements by going to a professional, but it makes it easier. Do the research on the companies; make sure they are at least GMP certified-and don't go by marketing testimonials.

Price is not always the determining factor for quality. Many of the cheaper supplements manufactured by the leading chain brands, are exactly what they advertise ... cheap. And some of the more expensive supplements are just that ... more expensive. They don't necessarily work either, so it's absolutely crucial that you're working with a professional, a health coach or someone who thoroughly understands nutrition and can teach you as you develop, grow and perform.

OMEGA-3 FATTY ACIDS IN GREATER DEPTH

Omega-3 fatty acids reduce inflammation and assist in cellular repair in the membrane that surrounds our cells (called the phospholipid bilayer). This membrane is actually two layers of fat, so this is where fat quality is extremely essential. When we break cells down, this layer allows for repairs that produce strong, intact, cell membranes that offer cell flexibility. It also provides cell permeability, for nutrients to get in and out properly as well as maintaining fluid balance in the cell. These are essential processes just to be a healthy person. As you increase the nutritional demands on your body by performance or through an injury it becomes even more critical.

Fish oil, avocados, nuts and seeds are going to be your main resources for Omega-3 fatty acids. Other oils, like olives, flaxseed, primrose, avocado and sesame oil are fantastic fatty acids and can actually help you lose weight.

FISH AS A SOURCE OF OMEGA-3 FATTY ACIDS

When looking for fish or fish oil, what you need are small, short-lived fish simply because the larger, ones that live longer naturally have more time to acquire more environmental toxins.

Almost all environmental toxins are fat-soluble. What are you taking when you take fish oil? Well, you're taking the fat of fish with fat-soluble, environmental toxins picked up from where they live. Therefore, smaller, younger fish are always going to be higher quality and provide a superior fish oil. When you are eating, you want to avoid farm-raised anything and larger fish, such as sword fish, that have had as many as ten or even twenty years to absorb and accumulate toxins in their fat.

PROTEIN

Proteins serve many functions within our bodies. I discuss this in an earlier section of this chapter. They help repair muscle tissue, but they are also required for immune system support. Proteins are involved in chemical reactions and amino acids are the building blocks to many different processes and tissues in our bodies that a good protein supplement can enhance for greater effectiveness.

Whey protein may seem to increase appetite but also elevates insulin. Post-exercise supplementation increases the rate of protein absorption. The Whey protein that I typically suggest is a CFM (cross flow micro-filtrated) isolate. This appears to offer the best availability to my patients with the least adverse effects.

I don't recommend taking in 45-50 grams of protein after high-intensity exercises because it puts a burden on your system to digest, absorb and utilize all of those amino acids at once. It can also be harmful to the kidneys. Several small meals at 20, 25, 30 grams of protein are best.

The average athlete should take post-workout supplementation within 45 minutes to an hour at the most, to increase the utilization of nutrients for repair and recovery. For intensity training and strength trainers, I suggest 1.5 grams of protein per kilogram of body weight.

BETA-ALANINE

Beta-Alaline does not appear to increase maximum strength, but it does improve short-term, high-intensity exercise. It delays fatigue and can be beneficial for short-distance sprinters, and swimmers. Beta-Alanine is an amino acid that works without any known harmful side effects. Few studies are done on Beta-Alanine, but it appears to be an effective and safe performance-enhancing supplement.

RIBOSE

Ribose is a sugar and is the component of RNA (a substance in the cells of plants and animals that helps make protein) in contrast to DNA. It appears to increase ATP (Energy) production at the cellular level. It is a worthwhile supplement to consider after a workout.

BCAA

BCAA stands for branched-chain amino acids. Leucine, in particular, when supplemented before and after exercise, appears to reduce muscle tissue damage and promote protein synthesis. One-third of muscle protein is comprised of BCAA's.

CREATINE

Creatine is a high-energy compound found in red meat and seafood. It is also synthesized by the pancreas, kidneys and liver. Creatine has been shown to promote rapid skeletal muscle regeneration of ATP, or energy, at a cellular level.

Oral Supplementation increases cellular Phosphocreatine concentrations from 15 to 40%. Creatine supplementation appears to be safe for strength and mass training. Increases in an athlete's size and mass appear to be attributed to cellular protein.

Creatine is a fascinating compound. It has been shown to regenerate the ADP, a phosphate donor to Adenosine Diphosphate, to Adenosine

Triphosphate, which is how you produce energy at a cellular level. The only clinical side effects are slight dehydration, cramping, some GI distress and weight gain.

If you want to be an elite athlete and increase one-rep max, muscle size and muscle strength, Creatine appears to be a high-quality supplement with minimal side effects to help achieve those goals.

HMB

HMB is [Beta] Hydroxymethylbutyrate acid. HMB is a metabolite of the essential amino acid, Leucine. More research is needed, however HMB appears to prevent the body from breaking down its proteins as fast, because the half-life of body protein and muscles is anywhere from 7 to 16 days. The research on this is a bit mixed, but it appears to have the effect of reducing the amount of muscle lost in between exercising.

L-CARNITINE

L-Carnitine helps to increase fatty-acid burning as fuel, and promotes muscle recovery. L-Carnitine, however, is somewhat controversial. A recent article published online in "Nature Medicine" indicated a possible link between L-Carnitine and atherosclerosis. I would anticipate continued research is appropriate, however, L-Carnitine does seem to be safe and effective. L-Carnitine increases the oxidation (burning) of fatty acids as fuel and aids in muscle recovery after intense exercise.

NITRIC OXIDE

Nitric Oxide is an Arginine product that enhances vasodilation during exercise due to Nitric Oxide synthesis. Vasodilation carries more blood to the muscles and, along with that, supplies more oxygen and nutrients. This increases the muscle's ability to produce more energy and appears to allow one to work out at an increased intensity.

Typically, you would take an Arginine product before working out. Taking even small amounts of L-Arginine significantly increases the Nitric

Oxide synthesis activity. It also appears to increase the vasodilation transport described earlier.

NUTRITION AND SPORTS PSYCHOLOGY

The brain is the organ in the body that is most nutrient and energy dependent; it is also the organ most vulnerable to toxins in our system. The higher the quality of fuel you give it to work the greater capacity the brain has to perform at its best. Considering your brain controls all voluntary and involuntary coordination throughout your entire body processes, your body can't be at peak performance if your brain is in a nutrient-poor environment.

Because the brain is so energy-dependent (or glucose-dependent, as I mentioned earlier), it's also vulnerable to the poisons in our body's waste elimination system. This is related to the toxic overload previously discussed.

Most athletes have the drive to succeed because they feed their brains well. If you give your brain high-quality fuel it can better control and coordinate the body's movement at a much higher capacity than if you're feeding it junk.

You want your brain to consume the highest quality fuel possible, so the higher quality nutrition you eat the better you perform.

What follows next are two lists of foods – the don'ts and the do's. These are very important to understand and follow as you build your strength and vitality through proper nutrition.

Do not eat

Ingredients:

Artificial Colors

Artificial Flavorings

Artificial Sweeteners: YES, I mean all of them!!!!!!!!

Benzoate Preservatives (BHT, BHA, TBHQ)

Brominated Vegetable Oil (BVO)

Carrageenan

Enriched Flours

High Fructose Corn Syrup (HFCS)

Maltodextrin

MSG (Monosodium Glutamate)

Olestra

Polysorbate 60

Propylene Glycol Alginate

Shortening, Hydrogenated and Partially Hydrogenated Oils:
(Palm, Soy bean and others)

Textured Soy Protein

These ingredients in their own way have been linked to dysfunction
Some examples are:

Allergies, Asthma, Dermatitis, Eczema, Hyperactivity, Headaches, Cancer,
Autoimmune Disorders, Digestive Disorders, Inflammatory Disorders,
Liver Disease, Kidney Disease, Fatigue, Obesity, Heart Disease, Stroke,
and many, many more.

**The list continues to grow. These are not the only food culprits,
however this is a good list to start the ball rolling.**

Food list

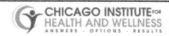

This is a list of high quality foods for your body. It is best when purchasing food that you look at the labels. It is important to buy mainly organic foods and to make sure that they are Non-GMO. Do not eat foods that you are allergic or sensitive to even if they are on this list.

Vegetables
- Spinach
- Arugula
- Asparagus
- Romaine Lettuce
- Leaf Lettuce
- Mushrooms
- Beets
- Cabbage
- Cucumbers
- Sweet Potato
- Onion
- Radish
- Artichokes
- Brussels Sprouts
- Kale
- Swiss Chard
- Bok Choy
- Parsnips
- Celery
- Carrots
- Leeks
- Shallot

Oils
- Olive
- Flax
- Avocado
- Coconut
- Sesame
- Apricot
- Safflower

Fruits
- Apples
- Avocado
- Plums
- Apricots
- Nectarines
- Cherries
- Mangos
- Currants
- Raspberries
- Blackberries
- Strawberries
- Cranberries
- Blueberries
- Prunes
- Figs
- Dates
- Pears
- Papaya
- Mango
- Lemons
- Limes

Beans
- Pinto
- Lima
- Garbanzo
- Butter
- Black

Meats
- Tuna
  (Water Packed)
- Salmon
- White Fish
  (All Varieties)
- Trout
- Turkey
- Chicken
- Beef (Limited)
- Pork (Limited)
- Eggs

Nuts & Seeds
- Sesame
- Cashews
- Pistachio
- Almonds
- Pumpkin
- Walnuts
- Filberts
- Pecans

Grains
- Quinoa
- Millet
- Amaranth
- Buckwheat
- Oats

Herbs & Spices
- Garlic
- Basil
- Cilantro
- Oregano
- Rosemary
- Thyme
- Bay Leaf
- Chives
- Caraway Seeds
- Curry
- Dill
- Cinnamon
- Dry Mustard
- Ginger
- Honey (Raw)
- Maple Syrup
- Rice Syrup
- Nutmeg
- Xanthan Gum
- Herbal Tea

Condiments
- Spike
- Liquid Aminos
- Sea Salt (Limited)
- Vinegar
- Apple Cider
  (Unfiltered w/the mother)

1750 N. Randall Rd. Suite 250 Elgin, IL 60123   Phone: 224-535-8707   Visit our Website: www.chicagohealthandwellness.com

Nutrition case study:

A 34 year-old female presented with anxiety and convulsive activity for over a year. She also stated that she would get whoozy during these episodes. She said the episodes started very infrequently, however they had been progressively getting worse in intensity and frequency. She had seen her primary care physician, endocrinologist, neurologist, rheumatologist and OB-GYN(none of whom could offer any answers or help) before walking into our clinic.

When evaluating her history we discovered that her 2 year-old daughter was breast feeding at a rate expected only from newborns (10-12 times per day). We also discovered that this woman was an avid exerciser that worked out daily - 6 to 7 times per week. During the exam, multiple signs of malnourishment and nutrient deficiencies were noticed in multiple systems of her body. We had run all of the necessary blood work, which all came out within the normal ranges, however most of the blood values were on the lower or higher side of normal.

Taking all of this information into consideration, we devised a plan of action which incorporated nearly every aspect of her lifestyle; diet, exercise, stress management, relaxation, sleep patterns, hormonal fluctuations, etc. We placed her on medical foods to supplement her nutritional status and modified her diet appropriately.

Six weeks into the program that we had laid out for her, she was completely asymptomatic. We were able keep her involved with exercise and her child continued to nurse for another full year without any issues.

Chapter 7

Health Coaching

WHAT ABOUT COACHING

Coaching at any level is an essential part of improving performance for all athletes. One of the best injury prevention practices an athlete can follow is to work with a sports-specific coach who is geared to the athlete's personal goals.

Every sports activity is technique driven. Throwing, catching, kicking, hitting a ball with your head or a bat are all technique-driven. Every sport that exists has coaches to help with techniques as well.

But, think about functions like standing, lifting, talking and walking. All are movements and poor movements lead to issues, both functional and structural.

A coach can help you by supplying you with the proper technique for the activity that you are to perform. This can certainly help prevent injuries and can increase your performance. All pros have professional sports coaches. Coaches exist in every sporting field and help athletes refine and fine tune performance to better the skill of athletes on their teams.

From personal experience, I feel strongly that proper coaching and injury prevention must begin before the high school or collegiate level. High schools, colleges and even early grade schools usually do not have the staff to coach athletes individually. Regardless, it's absolutely crucial that all young athletes be coached in the aspects of their lifestyles that impact their performance, including nutrition, training, and injury prevention.

It is rather ridiculous to believe that a young athlete can learn everything they need to know about being an athlete in a book or some pamphlets and apply it all on their own to become a champion.

ABOUT COACHES

All coaches are not created equal. It is indeed rare, in any profession, that all people involved in that profession are equal to one another. It is critically important that you have the right coach for you, no matter what your personality, motivation level, technical ability or deficiencies might be. You need a coach that is right for your level of commitment.

Make sure that the coach you choose matches your individual requirements. Also realize that as you grow and improve in your skills, your coaching needs will likely change.

WHAT KIND OF COACH DO YOU NEED

Do you need a swift kick in the pants to get going? Do you need congratulations and an "at a boy" at the end? Or, are you self-motivated and need only the technical aptitude as you strive ahead?

Different coaches bring different methodologies to the table. Based on your needs now and your abilities as you improve and play at a higher level, your coaching needs will undoubtedly change. Your coaches may need to change in the process.

Coaches tend to be extremely skilled in teaching technique, but each coach can be different in the techniques that they employ for the same sport. For example, if a pitcher were to go to five different pitching coaches, ranging in age from younger to older and more experienced, you would likely see five different methods (or more) to teach a pitcher how to throw better.

This diversity is great for the athlete because it affords him the opportunity to match his deficiencies in pitching with the proper coach for the job. And, it is like that in all sports. Greater diversity permits you as an athlete to find a coach tailored to work with your specific body mechanics/structure as well as your own individual sports "personality".

YOU MAY NOT KNOW WHAT YOU NEED IN A COACH!

Have you ever had an experience that made you uncomfortable, but a short while later not only was the discomfort gone, but you discovered something new about yourself that made you a better person? In general, working with a coach is like that. You might get a coach that is hard on you, or rides you, which makes you uncomfortable, resistant or frustrated. But, this approach might be the best thing for you.

YOU are the one that must recognize what works for you, what doesn't and be willing to make changes if needed. This is where the use of objective data comes into play.

COACHING AND OBJECTIVE DATA

I have a patient that was a high-level catcher on his high school baseball team, and he was looking to go to a Division 1 school. Unfortunately, he had issues in base running; essentially he was slightly slow on the bases. To improve, he went to a *speed camp* to work on those deficiencies. Sounds good… right?

I ran into him about a month after the camp was finished and asked, "Are you improving, running faster?"

"Yup", he said with confidence.

"Ok, what is your time in the 60 yard dash?" He gave me his answer and my next question was, "What was your time the first time you ran it?"

Answer: "I don't know, he never tested us initially."

BASELINES ARE VITAL TO KNOW PROGRESS

I guess you can't be wrong if you don't have a baseline to check progress against. This is obviously an isolated incident, but it does happen.

Coaches have access to all kinds of tools to assess athletes. These tools are essential to keep everyone accountable. Athletes need to practice and do the things they are asked to do. Consequently coaches need to modify what they are asking the athletes to do based upon the results. All of which is represented in objective data.

Numbers don't lie. I know that this is not totally true, however it is difficult to disagree with data. It is necessary to have bench marks and goals. More importantly, is to have the starting data to clearly show that you are on the right path to achieving your goals.

HEALTH COACHING

Health coaching is a special type of coaching using objective medical data to guide you in addressing and eliminating illness, disease, health conditions and to improve your energy levels for successful achievement of your goals. Health Coaching requires accountability of both the coach and the patient or athlete.

I think it's safe to say that everyone wants to be healthy but only a few really know how to get there. Health coaching is an educational process of learning from your health coach (who is an authority on a healthy living) and achieving your health goals. That is my definition. I am not saying that your health coach must be a physician because, quite frankly, I know some non-physicians that have an extensive, in-depth knowledge of the human organism.

FROM MY PERSPECTIVE

In my opinion, being a natural healthcare physician gives me a distinct advantage when it comes to working with all types of patients. Being a chiropractor gives me even more of an advantage. As a chiropractor, I have an in-depth, working knowledge of the mechanical (musculoskeletal system) portion of the human body. There are other healthcare professionals that also work with the body from a mechanical perspective, but a properly trained chiropractor has a thorough knowledge and understanding of the nervous system as well.

Chiropractors are Neuro-musculoskeletal specialists by definition. They intimately understand nerves, muscles, joints, bones and the biomechanics of the body (kinesiology). Integrating the nervous system into the treatment of a patient or into the performance of an athlete is critical.

The next advantage that I have, initially appears to be a disadvantage; NO DRUGS. In the state of Illinois, I can't prescribe medication. I think there are times when pharmaceuticals are necessary and I do feel that we are sufficiently trained to prescribe a certain class of pharmaceuticals. However, we do not have authority to do so.

Fortunately, this apparent "limitation" forces us to get to the bottom of health issues when helping people get better. We can't just give patients a prescription to make symptoms go away. Not having prescribing rights, allows us to determine the proper dietary plan, lifestyle modifications, supplement protocols, exercise regimens and stress relieving techniques customized to get that individual patient healthier from the inside, out.

This applies to athletes and dealing with performance issues as well. Like I've said many times, everyone is DIFFERENT, and when you use quantifiable, objective data as your guide to therapy, people get better.

It is tremendously gratifying to know that you played a bigger role than just making them feel better; you changed a patient's life.

Working with patients and athletes in this manner is difficult however. It requires meticulous record keeping, it's time consuming and it's an emotional investment in that individual that is not always 100% successful. You care deeply and it hurts when you don't hit that target.

Anything you do that has great, personal value to you is most likely difficult, and the sense of accomplishment that comes from watching a patient start to live their lives again far outweighs the strife.

HEALTH COACHING CASE STUDY

A 35 year-old female had been diagnosed with Lupus. She came to my office just before starting all the medications prescribed to subdue an out-of-control, inflammatory disease. She had three small children and one of the worst symptoms, included an inability to bend down and pick up her children due to pain. Her knees were swollen, painful and difficult to bend.

She had no energy at all, felt ill all the time and it was affecting her family relationship and dynamics.

We looked at her history and reports and made some pretty drastic changes to her lifestyle. We changed what she ate, drank, what kind of exercise she did, how much sleep she had at night and really worked on stabilizing her body's ability to handle stress.

Within the first 6 months, she was pain-free for the first time in years. She had energy again and patience with her children. Two years later she is totally symptom-free without medication. She lives the lifestyle that keeps her healthy and she does it with ease.

Now, she does full squats when she exercises without any knee issues what so ever and is still amazed at the feeling of squatting down with her kids. She is a superstar!

PROGRESSIVE OBJECTIVE TESTING

Health coaches, especially Sports Health Coaches, are invaluable to the athlete and non-athletes alike. I talked about coaches earlier and when they learn to use objective data, a Health Coach can truly shine. Most natural health care practitioners talk about having the ability to treat the whole person, but when you ask them how much lab work they run or how often they run it, you can often get a blank stare.

COACHES LEAVE YOUR EGOS AT THE DOOR

You must leave your ego at the door when working as a coach with patients. You have to accept the right to be wrong but always put forth your best effort. You must be adaptable to the patient's ever-changing requirements, not just what *you* think they need.

Health coaches often use numerous objective and verifiable tests when coaching our athletes or treating our patients. We test and retest to keep updated on their progress. This chapter covers some of the tests that are used in my practice, to demonstrate how these tools in health coaching can be used to improve performance. Below is a list of some of the most common tests we use:

- Bio-impedance Analysis
- Comprehensive Blood Work
- Hormone Panels
- Food and Environmental Allergy Testing
- Neurotransmitter Testing
- Allergy Testing
- Nutritional Evaluation Testing

WORKING WITH BODY IMPEDANCE ANALYSIS (BIA)

The Bio-Impedance Analysis (BIA), or body composition analysis, measures body composition electronically. This is the test we use to assess body fat, lean tissue density, fluid retention, hydration levels and cellular health. It's extremely valuable when you are placed on a detox/weight loss program because it gives you the accountability and feedback you need to be sure you are on the right track.

Report for JOHN DOE Tested on 14/09/2013 15:03:21

Body Composition Report created by

Chicago Institute for Health & Wellness
1750 N. Randall Rd. Suite 250
Elgin, IL 60123
224-535-8707

BIA Results:	Male	Name:	JOHN DOE
Height in:	72	Date:	Monday, 16 September 2013 13:36:53
Weight lb:	200	Database:	C:/ProgramData/RJL Systems/BC/Databases//Patients.db
Age:	40	Subject ID:	
Chosen Goal Wt.	178.0 lb	Record date:	14/09/2013 15:03:21
BMI:	27.12	Equation Set:	Athletic
Resistance:	432	Reactance:	70 ohms
Phase angle:	9.2	Impedance:	437.6

	Date: 14-Sep-13
Height (in):	72.00
Weight (lb):	200.00
Age:	40
Resistance:	432.0
Reactance:	70.0
Actual BMI:	27.12
Actual phase:	9.2
Estimated BMR:	1960
% ideal FAT:	17.6
% estimated FAT:	17.9
Wt estimated FAT:	35.9
% estimated FFM:	82.1
Wt estimated FFM:	164.1
% estimated LDM:	24.9
Wt estimated LDM:	49.8
% WT estimated TBW:	57.2
Liters estimated TBW:	51.8
% TBW estimated ICW:	57.9
Liters estimated ICW:	30.0
% TBW estimated ECW:	42.1
Liters estimated ECW:	21.8

The Bio-Impedance Analysis is a tissue and fluid test. When there is a normal distribution of tissue and fluid within the body, it indicates a high level of immunity, a high functional level and good longevity.

If I see an abnormal distribution of tissue and fluid, it indicates susceptibility and low function which can impact the natural healing processes and cause premature aging.

IS THIS THE END-ALL, BE-ALL TEST

Not really, because it has a tiny margin of error. However, this is a clinically significant, objective, reproducible, easy to perform examination and it allows us to compare data set to data set each time we see a patient. This is a very easy procedure compared to the impracticality of running blood work on patients weekly or bi-monthly.

Consider your body as bioelectric. That means there is an electrical current that flows through your body tissues. Body Bio-Impedance Analysis measures your vitality at a cellular level.

The machine that we use in the office measures the following:

- Phase Angle
- Body Capacitance
- Resistance
- Reactance
- Body Cell Mass
- Extracellular Mass
- Fat-Free Mass
- Fat Mass
- Extracellular Mass to Body Cell Mass Ratio
- Body Mass Index
- Basal Metabolic rate
- Intracellular Water

- Extracellular Water
- Total Body Water
- Total Body Water to Fat-Free Mass Ratio
- Total Body Water to Total Weight Ratio

The phase angle is concerned with cellular health and integrity, and is based upon research demonstrating a relationship between phase angles. Cellular health is increasing and nearly linear. When I see a low phase angle, it indicates that the cell is unable to store energy, and therefore breaks down in the selective permeability of cellular membranes.

The angle gives you an indication of the cell lipid status because cell membranes have such a high lipid content. If the indicator shows a high phase angle, this signals to me that there are large quantities of intact, healthy cell membranes and a high body cell mass.

The phase angle values for adults usually range from 3 to 10 degrees, and a normal value generally falls between 6 to 8 degrees. If I see a value 5 degrees or less, this can mean there is a serious energy deficiency. I try to push my patients into the area of 8 degrees or higher.

A resistance value is the ratio of electrical potential to the current in a material. Water is a great conductor of electricity and would, therefore, have a low resistance. By contrast, rubber has a high resistance and, therefore, conducts poorly. As I just mentioned, water is the main conductor in the body, so if there is a low-resistance value that usually indicates that the patient's body has a high percentage of lean body mass. The opposite is also true; a high resistance score means there are lower amounts of lean body mass.

Resistance helps to calculate the amount of water in the body. Low resistance, indicating high conductivity, is due to large amounts of water in the body. Resistance in the body is proportional to the amount of lean body mass since water is contained solely within lean body mass.

The next measurement is reactance, which is the cells' ability to store energy. High reactance means that the body stores energy easily. A body that stores energy poorly has low reactance. The BIA measures the energy that is stored in the cell membrane. This measure gives an indication of the amount of intact cell membranes throughout the body. The reactance of the body is proportional to the amount of body cell mass. This is a crucial measure as it relates to the proportion of the body that is metabolically active.

Another measure that the BIA performs is lean body mass or fat-free mass. This is a measure of the total amount of nonfat (lean) body parts. Lean body mass consists of about 73% water, 20% protein, 6% mineral, and 1% ash. In the lean body mass most of the body's water (all the metabolically active tissues and bone) is the source of all metabolic caloric expenditure.

What remains is called the fat mass, which contains all the extractable lipids from adipose and other tissues in the body. Simply put, this is your body fat. This is a measure of the total amount of stored lipids (fats) in the body and consists of subcutaneous fat and visceral fat. Subcutaneous fat is located directly beneath the skin and serves as an energy reserve and as insulation against outside cold. Visceral fat is located deeper within the body and serves as an energy reserve and as a cushion between organs. You cannot live without some fat in your body. The ideal amount depends on a person's age and gender.

The number of calories consumed and metabolized at a resting state over 24 hours is called the Basal Metabolism Rate or BMR. For many of my patients, the BMR accounts for more than 90% of their total daily expenditure. The reason is that more than 90% of calories are burned while they are at rest.

The BMR is determined by lean body mass, since only lean body mass metabolizes. The BMR is higher in connection to the lean body mass. One of the main benefits of exercise is the maintenance of lean body mass.

You can consume fewer calories and reduce the lean body mass, which may negatively affect the body's ability to burn calories. My job includes helping my patients build leaner body mass as this reduces and maintains weight.

When you are losing weight, building lean body mass is hard, so I concentrate on helping them minimize its reduction. Consider that a typical patient will lose 0.45 pounds of lean body mass and 0.55 pounds of fat mass for each pound of weight loss if they lose weight without exercising and concentrate only on their diet.

A person's Body Mass Index or BMI is a measure of a person's weight relative to their height, and while this can be done with a calculator, the BIA does it for me.

The BIA also calculates Total Body Water. Remember, as I mentioned earlier, most of the water in the body is contained in lean body mass. The Total Body Water calculation takes into account Intracellular Water (ICW) and Extracellular Water (ECW). This is an important calculation because it indicates a client's basic hydration status.

THE ICW is a measure of the water inside a cell. If the cells are healthy, they will hold water easily within the cell membrane. This water inside the cell is necessary to retain water-soluble nutrients such as vitamins B and C. The target number for ICW depends on gender and age, but generally, 2/3 of your water should be inside the cell.

The ECW is the water outside the cell. This water is necessary to retain some nutrients and helps to expel waste from inside the cell. This is the remaining 1/3 of your Total Body Water. When I see a low ICW, this can mean dehydration, nutritional imbalance, hormonal imbalance or toxicity.

The percentage of lean body mass that is water is also calculated by the BIA. I look for values around 73% of fat-free mass that is water. Another percentage that is calculated is the total weight that is water. For men, it is about 60% and for women about 55%. Again, these values give me information about hydration, cell health and the body's energy level.

Once I do my initial BIA assessment, I continue to recheck each time a client comes into the office. This helps track patient progress through objective data. As a patient begins to increase their physical activities, the BIA should demonstrate an increase in lean body mass, body cell mass and phase angle. Using these numbers, I am able to help my client manage their diet and nutrition and their exercise program, which leads to the overall improvement of their physical condition.

EXPLAINING THE BIA AND HOW IT WORKS

The BIA has two main cable leads and each of the leads has two crocodile/alligator clips; a red and a black. I attach these clips to the exposed tabs on the electrodes. I then enter information such as the client's Gender, Age, Height, Weight, Activity Level and Waist/Hip measurements using the three keypads.

Once this data is entered, the BIA unit passes a safe, battery-generated signal through the body so that it can measure the bioelectrical impedance at a fixed frequency of 50kHz. When completed, the BIA displays a complete body composition analysis in the areas I already mentioned: Body Fat, Lean Body Mass, Total Body Water, optimal ranges, metabolic rates, BMI and Waist/Hip Ratios.

BLOOD PANELS, NUTRITION, ALLERGY AND HORMONE LEVEL TESTS

ALLERGY TESTS

Another test we can perform is a quick blood analysis to determine things you might be allergic to, including substances that are airborne, food-related and environmental allergens (including regional allergens). It's a fast test with quick results.

Knowing what you are allergic to is vital so that we can create a plan that might include an avoidance diet. Understanding that everyone's body doesn't react the same way to each allergen, makes it necessary to test for not just a histamine reaction (typical reaction of hives, itching, swollen eye, etc.) but to also test for an inflammatory reaction. Chronic inflammation to athletes and non-athletes alike is the bane of our existence.

Allergy panels test for:

- Molds
- Grasses, Trees, Weeds and Fungi
- Gluten Intolerance
- Foods
- Functional Foods and Herbs
- Food Additives/Colorings
- Environmental Chemicals
- Pediatric Allergy Panel

COMPLETE BLOOD COUNT (CBC WITH DIFF./PLATELET)

At our clinic we do a Complete Blood Count, or CBC, as this will give me a decent idea of your overall health. The results give me information about the kinds and the number of cells in your blood.

CHEMISTRY PANEL (16 ESSENTIAL TESTS)

Another useful test is the Chemistry Panel of 16 essential tests that provides another quick snapshot of your overall health. This type of test requires the patient to fast for at least 12 hours prior to the blood test to be sure that the results are accurate.

CHOLESTEROL BLOOD TEST (LIPIDS WITH HDL/LDL RATIO)

The Cholesterol blood test gives me a clear picture of whether you have abnormal cholesterol or triglyceride levels. High levels may indicate a higher risk for heart disease or other coronary (heart) illnesses. In some cases, we may refer the patient back to their primary care giver or specialist. We can also easily develop a diet and exercise program within our own clinic that can improve these numbers.

Another test we can order is a VAP® Cholesterol Test. This is a more comprehensive panel that reports on 18 separate components of blood cholesterol compared to just four in a standard test.

MICRONUTRIENT TEST

Whenever I work with a patient and nutrition, I feel that I'd better get to know what is going on nutritionally with them as this impacts their metabolic processes and how fast they heal. One test we perform is a MicroNutrient test. This one determines the body's ability to absorb 32 vitamins, minerals, antioxidants and other essential nutrients within the white blood cells. Once we know what the body is deficient in, we help the patient create a nutrition plan to increase those nutrients in their diet or through adding supplements.

NEUROTRANSMITTER TESTING

Neurotransmitters are natural brain chemicals that your brain uses to function. These are manipulated when using pharmaceuticals for depression, anxiety, and attention deficit disorders. Although you would think that these tests should be done to learn the nature of the chemical imbalance in the patients being prescribed these drugs, this test is almost never done *before* medication begins.

We test these brain chemicals regularly, simply because we are looking for root causes. If there is a chemical imbalance, it is necessary to treat appropriately and sometimes that means pharmaceuticals, although many times it does not. Anti-depressive drug prescriptions are growing at an alarming rate and are in the top five drugs prescribed in America. When did we become so imbalanced?

Essentially, we take pills to feel better about feeling bad. My suggestion is to look at the alternatives, work on improving your health and you will be amazed at how much better you feel in a remarkably short period of time, through more natural methods.

HORMONE TESTING

We offer several different hormone tests, but I am partial to saliva testing as it measures your hormones throughout the day. Our hormone levels change during our lives, and they can change significantly, even in the course of a single day. Some are higher in the morning, some at night. This test can help show a true picture of your hormones and what is going on with you during the entire day.

Hormone levels have an affect on many aspects of our bodies, both emotionally and physically. Included in these aspects are irritability, weight gain, memory lapses, insomnia, depression and fatigue.

Blood tests for hormones provide a small amount of information at one point in time. We offer a comprehensive hormone health panel, which is a saliva hormone test and includes Testosterone, Progesterone, Estradiol, DHEA, Cortisol, and Melatonin.

MEN'S HEALTH

We also offer a number of tests specifically for men and women. Each gender has particular issues that can specifically impact them. We test for different elements, and the test results also have distinctive ranges dependent on gender.

When a man has a hormone imbalance, he might suffer from fatigue, headache, weight gain, irritability, infertility, mood swings, loss of libido (sex drive) and depression.

It is an excellent idea for all men to be checked, head to foot, for wellness at least once a year, or before they begin to engage in any new exercise program, diet or sport. Our clinic offers a Comprehensive Male Panel, which gives us a look at everything that's in the Basic Checkup panel, but includes male-specific items such as the PSA, Testosterone, and DHEA–S tests. All of these results can help me develop individualized plans for fertility, libido, and increased muscle mass.

DHEA–S (Dehydroepiandrosterone Sulfate)

Your adrenal glands are located on top of each of your kidneys and produce and release certain regulatory hormones and chemical messengers. One is Dehydroepiandrosterone Sulfate or DHEA–S. This is a natural steroid hormone produced from cholesterol, and its purpose is to serve as a component of male and female sex hormones. This hormone is also associated with the immune and stress response.

TESTOSTERONE (FREE, DIRECT, WITH TOTAL)

Testosterone is the hormone found in men and women but is generally much higher in men. It affects sexual features and development. Testosterone levels are the highest after puberty and will continue to rise until a man reaches 40 years of age. The decreased levels of testosterone have been found to lead to significant lowering of libido and athletic performance levels.

WOMEN'S HEALTH

Likewise, our clinic offers a specific Comprehensive Female Panel that will determine if your hormones are functioning properly. In addition to what is in the Basic Check–Up panel, we include Estradiol, LH, Progesterone, FSH, and DHEA–S tests.

ESTRADIOL

This is similar to the testosterone test in men as it tests the amount of estradiol (a form of estrogen) in your blood. This helps me assess your estrogen status, which helps in understanding your ovarian function and monitoring the follicular development during ovulation. There are also instances in which I may perform this test on men to assess their estrogen production levels.

These are just a few of the tests that can be performed by a health coach, and are essential in determining what the individual needs are for a particular athlete or patient. Utilizing the data, the coach can then create a comprehensive program. This is NOT something that an athlete can (or should) attempt on his or her own.

Case study:

A 26 year-old female patient presented with anxiety, weight issues, fatigue, fogginess, allergies, chronic headaches and neck pain. She indicated that she had a high-stress job in the retail environment, and that she was burnt out with her position and health status. She was ready to feel better.

We did our usual comprehensive medical work-up and discovered multiple issues that we addressed with structural manipulation and nutritional guidance. She proceeded to get healthier, feel better, get some clarity of thought and get her energy levels back.

One of the things that she indicated early was that she was an artist, loved photography, but always hated school. She was incredibly sharp and had a fantastic business mind, which is why she managed retail, but again did not like her position. So, I very simply asked her, "Now that you have your life back, what are you going to do with it?" It was a simple question, but for the first time in years she had the health and energy to think about it.

Within 3 months, she applied to and was accepted at one of the top schools in the country, where she started her bachelors' degree in photography. Needless to say, we are all very proud of her! You never know where life leads until you have the health and energy to fully engage in it.

Concluding Notes

I am confident that this book has given you a fair amount of understanding about general health, nutrition, physical exercises, etc., and also enough insight about various sports injuries and preventive tips.

Now it's up to you. Let me end this book with an acronym for life:

BE HEALTHY

Be Engaged: Pay attention to your body and to the world around you

Eating: Certain Foods are inflammatory:

Stay away from

Wheat, Dairy, Eggs, Corn, Sugar, Sugar Substitutes, processed foods, caffeine, NO SODA

Try this for a two weeks and see how you feel. You may not notice in the first couple of days but you would be amazed at the difference in the way you feel in two weeks. Give it time and you will feel a night and day difference.

Habits: Set your routine: We are creatures of habit, so make them good ones

Elimination: This pertains to metabolic waste as well as toxic aspects of your life, such as relationships, work environments, and excuses: There are a million excuses for why we can't do something, but none of them are as good as the reason to do it

Activity: Stay in motion: We are not meant to be sedentary so get your butt moving! It doesn't have to be 30 min 3X per week but it is about the discipline to stay in motion; conditioning will come with this habit

Liquids: This means water: Caffeine, juice, soda, alcohol do not count. Stay Hydrated:

Thinking: Link your thinking to your actions and your actions to your thinking:

i. Your body's patterns of behavior are linked to the way you think and the opposite is also true.

ii. If you're not feeling great that day, go do something that makes you feel great, ie: hobbies, exercise or reading read a fun book

Heal: Let your body heal and rest. Take the necessary time off and take the time to rehab an injury correctly. Jumping back in too soon only leads to further injuries and less productive performance. Don't forget to get enough sleep: Sleep is the time when your body heals

Y: "Why" & Comply

1. Don't just accept that you have an issue; ask yourself and your doctor why is this happening and what are we doing that is causing/has caused health issues to occur.

2. If you don't get a satisfactory answer, fire your doctor! "Satisfactory" does not mean the answer you *want* to hear, by the way.

3. Comply! Once you have received your answers, follow through with the prescribed treatment plan. That is your obligation as the patient.

Index

Made in the USA
Monee, IL
08 July 2021

73179826R00089